CATARACTS

Cataracts: What You Must Know About Them

Charles D. Kelman, M.D.

CROWN PUBLISHERS, INC.
NEW YORK

This book is dedicated to
my father and mother,
who said, "First be a doctor."

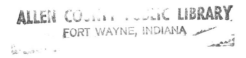
Copyright © 1982 by Charles D. Kelman, M.D.

All rights reserved. No part of this book may be reproduced or
transmitted in any form or by any means, electronic or mechanical,
including photocopying, recording, or by any information storage and
retrieval system, without permission in writing from the publisher.

Published by Crown Publishers, Inc.,
One Park Avenue, New York, New York 10016, and simultaneously in
Canada by General Publishing Company Limited

Manufactured in the United States of America

Library of Congress Cataloging in Publication Data

Kelman, Charles D.
Cataracts : what you must know about them.

Includes index.
1. Cataract—Surgery. I. Title.
RE451.K367 1982   617.7'42059   82-9771
ISBN: 0-517-54850-X   AACR2
10 9 8 7 6 5 4 3 2 1

FIRST EDITION

2074212

Contents

Photographs follow page 22

Foreword

In the early 1970s, I, like all ophthalmologists around the world, began to read in medical journals and learn at medical meetings of a marvelous new way of cataract removal invented by Dr. Charles Kelman of New York City. So revolutionary, and with such quick and wonderful recovery of vision, the method could not help but attract the attention of the news media—often stimulated by excited and grateful patients. I began to learn the method together with one of the earliest Kelman machines, and realized it was the way I could help most of my cataract patients.

During this time, it was my happy privilege to take my family down the Colorado River on a rubber raft, and during the five-day trip, I realized that those little blurry flecks were not on the beautiful red walls, but instead were some kind of defects within my own eyes.

At Las Vegas, a former ophthalmology resident kindly undertook a late-night examination and confirmed that I—in my early sixties—was developing a cataract in each eye. My sight rapidly failed, my nondominant eye first. Although I knew on a first-name basis almost every well-known eye surgeon in the world, it was obvious that I would prefer to have Dr. Kelman. My recovery after his surgery was phenomenal. Ten days after I myself had been operated on, I operated on the eyelids of the late Colonel Harland Sanders of Kentucky Fried Chicken fame. The

Colonel was so pleased that he made a donation of $200,000 to the Eye Foundation Hospital in Birmingham, Alabama!

Now nearly ten years have elapsed since my first cataract operation. At that time I obtained soft contact lenses; now I would have implant lenses, since they have been perfected—Dr. Kelman's implant lenses being outstanding. But the fact is that I now have been a productive surgeon for ten years since my cataract surgery. I am one of more than twelve thousand grateful Kelman patients.

ALSTON CALLAHAN, M. D.

Preface

You are sitting in the examining chair. The room is almost dark, and it is quiet.

You are hoping for the best, but you are prepared for the worst. Yet, when the words come, somehow you still are not prepared. You hold on tight to the arm of the chair and your knuckles whiten.

"You have a cataract," says the doctor.

"A cataract," you whisper. "Oh, my God."

Images of blindness . . . old age . . . Seeing Eye dogs . . . all appear before your cataract-filled eyes. You hold on tighter to the armrest. It's all you can do not to shriek, "Take it out! Quick! Before it spreads!"

Meanwhile, the doctor is explaining a few things to you, but your mind goes blank. The images start reappearing and they are getting worse: things you have to do but now cannot; things you want to do but will never be able to do again.

You work yourself up to such a pitch that before you know it, you are handing back to the doctor's nurse a form authorizing surgery, without even having read it.

Later, when you have had time to let it all sink in, you realize that you have a million unanswered questions on your mind.

Like: "My God, what will happen if something goes wrong?" "Do I really need this?" "Can't I wait?" "Is he the right doctor to do it?" "Can I trust this guy with my eyes?" "Should I get another opinion?" "Why me, why me?" and, of course, "Will I go blind?"

Now is the time to sit down and to be calm.

Don't be so tough on yourself. Chances are that even if you had kept yourself under control, you would not have thought of all the questions at once. As a matter of fact, you probably would not even have known the right questions to ask.

So relax. This book will answer all your questions, and then some. It will make you aware of those questions you should ask and why you should ask them. It will tell you what to do if you do not get the right answers.

It will tell you what the right answers are because, after all, you have the right to know.

Most of all, it will help put your mind at rest—and put your precious eyes in the hands of the surgeon who is right for you.

1

Choosing Your Surgeon

If you suspect that you have a cataract, the first thing you must do is consult an ophthalmologist (see the Glossary at the end of this book). Then, if you feel that you need a cataract operation, you should check on your ophthalmologist's credentials.

First, check on whether he has been certified, and is a fellow of, the American Academy of Ophthalmology. If he is certified, he has passed an extremely difficult series of examinations about the structure, function, and diseases of the eye. This attests to his knowledge only, not to his skill or his approach. If he is a fellow, he passed.

Also ask some patients of his in the waiting room how they were referred. If from another doctor, that is one thing. If they all read newspaper articles about him, that is entirely another.

If you have no ophthalmologist and suspect or have been told that you have cataracts, call your local medical society or use the list of local ophthalmology associations at the end of this book. There you will get several names from which to choose.

Here is how inquiries are handled by them, all according to proper ethical standards.

In 1970, after I had developed the technique of phacoemulsification (see the Glossary), many unsolicited newspaper articles were written about it. Subsequently,

1

when patients called the medical societies, they were told, and rightly so, that this was something new, something perhaps not yet totally proved, but an actual new technique. Now the operation is of course widely accepted.

Today, however, because of the Supreme Court ruling allowing professionals to advertise, many people are taken in by printed stories of a few doctors who imply that they are using new techniques. I have seen some of those stories, and I can vouchsafe to you that the techniques have been around for at least fifteen years.

So, if you happen to read one of these articles or hear a report of a "new technique," put in a call to your local medical society to confirm what you have read, or to straighten out the facts. You may well be spared a visit to the office of a physician who has implied to the newspapers that his skill is greater than it actually is.

On the other hand, if the society informs you that it is indeed a new procedure, you may want to ask how to secure some printed information about it. Or you may write to the doctor himself and ask for further information. If the "new" technique has not been reported in a recognized scientific journal, forget about it—and about him.

Obtaining a Second Opinion

If you suspect that you have a slight decrease in your vision and your ophthalmologist confirms this and tells you that you do have a cataract but that it does not require surgery, a second opinion is unnecessary. Your ophthalmologist is being totally honest with you, as most of them are. He is not prepared to do unnecessary surgery.

If you are not in distress about your vision, just go back and see this doctor regularly, whenever he recommends that you do so. You can have confidence in him.

Suppose you have been seeing an ophthalmologist for years and he has been following your cataract. Now you are seeing poorly and he tells you that surgery is required. In this instance also a second opinion is not necessary.

If, on the other hand, you have minimal visual distress,

and an ophthalmologist tells you that you have a cataract requiring surgery, a second opinion is advisable.

When you go to a doctor for a second opinion, it is important that you go in cold. Do not tell him about the previous diagnosis, and do not give the previous recommendation. Let the doctor start afresh, without being biased.

If the second doctor agrees with the first and tells you, "Yes, you do have a cataract, and yes, it does require surgery," then I suggest you have it—but only if your life-style has been adversely affected. And to have the operation, you should return to the ophthalmologist with whom you are most familiar.

In seeking a second opinion, the reason you do not reveal that the first doctor suggested an operation is in case you happen to come upon one of those rare specialists who are looking for more business. This insidious game, which, fortunately, only a very few ophthalmologists practice, goes as follows:

Dr. A. correctly recommends surgery for one of his patients. The patient goes for a second opinion to Dr. B. Dr. B. knows that Dr. A. recommended surgery and says to the patient, "You do not need an operation at this time. You may never need an operation. Dr. A. was wrong in recommending it. Come back and see me in six months."

The patient loses confidence in Dr. A. Six months later when he goes back to Dr. B., the doctor says, "Well, now you are ready for cataract surgery, and I'll be happy to do it."

This is why it is important that you not tell your second-opinion doctor what the first doctor recommended, particularly if you got the second doctor's name from a newspaper story.

The worst kind of second-opinion consultation you can get is a long-distance one. If you live in California and have heard of a New York doctor who is an excellent cataract surgeon, by all means do not, and I repeat, do not, go to New York for your surgery, for the following reason:

Even after successful cataract surgery, a certain amount of postoperative care is required. In most cases, it is minimal. But in some cases, even with a good result, several visits are required, for changes in medication and careful follow-up. In complicated cases, even more follow-up is necessary.

If you have a long-distance surgeon and are anxious to get back home, you may well compromise the outcome of your surgery. Even months later you may need some special attention, such as for an eroding suture (stitch) that must be removed. If you then call your local ophthalmologist, he will be rightly indignant that you did not come to him for the surgery, and he may or may not be willing to see you. Although you will probably eventually find someone to take care of you, you will most likely not be so well served, or in the same spirit, as you would have been had you had the surgery locally.

I repeat: Do not travel more than a hundred miles for your operation if there is someone locally who is equipped to do it.

If you have a special type of cataract, requiring special equipment and techniques, chances are that your local ophthalmologist will be only too glad to refer you to someone specialized in that technique. In that case, it is good to travel to that specialist. And in that case, your local ophthalmologist will be happy to follow you postoperatively.

If you get diametrically opposing opinions from two ophthalmologists, then you can probably go along with the opinion that suits you more. For example, one specialist tells you that you do not need cataract surgery and another says that you do. If you feel comfortable with the vision you have, follow the recommendation of the doctor who advises against operating; if not, follow the other's. Or suppose you decide that you really do need surgery to improve your way of life, and one ophthalmologist feels he should not operate yet, but another thinks he can. Unless there is some complicating disease, you might well allow the willing surgeon to operate.

Another alternative is to get still a third opinion. The need for this is very rare, and if you are going to get a third opinion, it is best to inform the doctor that you are there only for an opinion, not for surgery, even if he should recommend it. Whichever of the first two surgeons he agrees with, you may go along with.

If all this sounds confusing to you, you must remember that medicine is not a science. Surgery is not a science. There are no medical situations that are simply black or white. We are dealing with an art—the art of healing and the art of surgery. Just as you might go to two very competent artists for your portrait and each picture would look entirely different, so it is with surgeons. Each one operates from his background of experience and abilities. There are no absolutes.

2

What Is a Cataract?

Before we go any further, I would like to give you a mini-course in the components of your eye. This will help you to understand better what is going on when we discuss cataract development.

Although it is an old one by now, the analogy between a camera and the human eye is a good one.

The camera has an external lens. You can see this readily by looking at a camera and watching the light reflecting off the front surface of the lens.

In your eye, there is also an external lens (see figure 1a). You can see this lens if you look in a mirror and shine a light on your eye. You will see the light reflecting off your external lens. The only difference is that in the human eye this structure is not called a lens, it is called the cornea.

The cornea of the eye and the external lens of the camera both serve to partly focus the light.

If you try to touch your own external lens, the cornea, you will find it very difficult to do. The cornea is extremely sensitive. Although there are no blood vessels in it (and that is why it is clear), it has more nerves in it than most tissues in the body. This is, of course, a protective mechanism.

Now, back to your camera. It may have a dial that you can turn to open and close a diaphragm. This controls the amount of light allowed in.

In the eye, this diaphragm is called the iris (see figure 1b). It is the colored portion of the eye—usually blue or brown. If you stand in a semidarkened room and look in a mirror while shining a light into your eye, you will see the pupil rapidly get smaller. This iris tissue is rapidly and constantly moving, adjusting the amount of light let into the eye. Later on, in Chapter 8, when we talk about the positioning of implants, we will see why it is important that an implant not be in contact with your rapidly moving iris.

Now let us talk about what is behind your iris. If your camera is equipped with a lens that can be unscrewed, you can take out the lens and discover that there is more than one. There is a rear lens. Behind the iris in your eye there is also a rear lens (see figure 1c). (Remember that your front lens was called the cornea.) The rear lens is sometimes called the crystalline lens. Indeed, that is the subject of this book: the crystalline lens of the eye that has become clouded.

Your crystalline lens is slightly smaller than a lima bean. It is perfectly clear, like glass, and in its normal state is colorless. What it does is to fine-focus the light that was partially focused by the outer lens, the cornea.

The shape of your lens automatically changes when you want to look to a distance, or when you want to look close up. The closer you focus, the more spherical or round the lens becomes. This marvelous focusing is accomplished by muscles that surround the lens. These muscles contract and relax, pulling or relaxing the tension of the ligaments (zonules) that hold the lens in place (see figure 1d).

Sometimes I wonder how the most confirmed atheist can deny the presence of a deity in the face of such an ingenious design as that of the human eye!

The ligaments that hold the lens and allow it to adjust its shape also serve another important function. They hold back the jelly (the vitreous humor) that is behind the lens (see figure 1e) and keep it from entering the front portion of the eye.

The retina of your eye is like the film in your camera (see figure 1f). What keeps this retina in place is the jelly behind your lens. Retinal detachment will be discussed in Chapter 6.

As I said, your lens is normally clear, and it is always changing its shape—practically every second of the day. And sometimes, due to usage or age or other causes, it begins to yellow. This is the beginning of a cataract.

That's what a cataract is: simply a darkening, a change in color from clear to yellow to brown and, finally, to black or opaque. Only when the lens has become totally opaque does the patient become totally blind. We call that opacification, from the word *opaque*.

The time that it takes for opacification varies. Usually, from the first sign of yellowing to the time when the patient can no longer adequately see from the eye is a period of many, many years, often decades.

To understand why this change in the lens takes place, we must go back a bit. There are no blood vessels in your transparent crystalline lens, just as there are none in the cornea. Blood vessels, which nourish other parts of the body, would not allow light to pass. So in order to get nourishment, the lens is bathed in a nutrient fluid called the aqueous humor (see figure 1). Sometimes this nourishment is insufficient. If so, after a long time the lens begins to change color and gradually forms a cataract. Such cataracts are often called senile cataracts. This name actually has nothing to do with senility, or the loss of mental or other faculties. It merely implies that it comes with age.

We have not been successful, at this point in science, in significantly retarding the aging process. But I believe—although it has not been scientifically substantiated—that since vitamin C plays a role in the metabolism of the lens, taken in slightly larger than normal doses, vitamin C could conceivably retard the formation of cataracts.

Again—and this is not a scientific recommendation—I suggest to some patients with beginning cataracts that they take anywhere from one thousand to two thousand milligrams a day of ascorbic acid (vitamin C).

As to what else causes cataracts, light—especially ultraviolet light and infrared (heat) light—is implicated in some cases. For instance, there is the well-known "glass-blower's cataract," which comes from being exposed to high-intensity heat. In these cases, it is suspected that the infrared rays, the hot rays, are causing the protein of the lens to degenerate.

There are other types of cataracts besides the senile one. Infants can, in fact, get cataracts. They can be born with them, or they can develop them at a very early age. These cataracts usually are hereditary when there is a genetic disturbance that affected the development of the lens. Sometimes trauma can cause children's cataracts also.

A cataract in a baby is an emergency, because it has been shown that the very first months, weeks, and even days are crucial for the development of connections between the eye and the brain. As a matter of fact, monkeys that are blindfolded from birth and later have the blindfold removed at differing times, are unable to discern small objects. If the blindfold has been left on for more than six months, they become practically blind. Certainly, a child's eye that has been blinded by cataracts up to the age of more than five or six years can no longer be made to see adequately, even if the cataract is then removed.

The diagnosis of a congenital cataract can usually be made by a pediatrician looking into the child's eye immediately at birth. An alert mother can sometimes notice a cataract by simply looking at the normally black pupil. If is is white instead, an immediate visit to an ophthalmic surgeon is indicated. If the cataract is visible to the mother, then it probably is well developed and surgery is indicated immediately.

While most ophthalmologists are used to dealing with senile cataracts, not all are totally experienced with infant ones. So, in line with what was said in Chapter 1, if you have a child with a cataract, ask your doctor how many cataracts he has removed from children. If you and/or he feels that he is not experienced enough to deal with this situation, have him refer you to someone who is. This is a highly specialized operation, requiring highly specialized equipment.

Another type of cataract is one that is caused by certain medications. For example, it is known that cortisone taken over a long period will cause a cataract on the posterior layer of the lens.

Certain other medications are also cataractogenic, or cataract causing. There is the possibility that certain strong medications used to treat glaucoma are a cause, because we have noticed a predisposition of patients who have been on long-standing glaucoma medications to get cataracts later on.

Also responsible for cataracts are exposures to high doses of X-ray radiation and high-frequency sonar waves. This is why the sonar ovens require careful monitoring for leaks.

SEE NOTE BELOW

Certain diseases, such as diabetes, retinitis pigmentosa, and others, also can cause cataracts at an age earlier than is common.

Trauma is another cause of cataracts. Any penetrating instrument, such as a knife or ice pick, can be a cause, as can a severe dull blow. Many boxers develop cataracts this way, particularly if they have been exposed to dirty fighting, like punches to the eye with the thumb of the boxing glove.

Now that you are familiar with the physiology of your eye and some of the causes of cataracts, let us discuss some of the symptoms.

Let me stop here, however, and say that although you may suspect that you are suffering from some of these symptoms, you must have the diagnosis confirmed by an ophthalmologist. This may sound silly to you, but there are a lot of people who start to have symptoms of diseases merely through the power of suggestion. Or you might have some other condition requiring treatment.

When a person develops a cataract, the first thing he notices is a darkening of his vision. Or, if you have what we call a posterior cataract, you may notice that when you are out in bright lights, the glare affects you, or, when you are driving at night and a headlight shines directly into your eye, you are temporarily blinded.

The darkening of the vision is due to a yellowing of the

NOTE RE "SONAR" & MORE LIKELY "RADAR", THAT IS, MICRO-WAVE OVENS NOW COMMON IN KITCHENS.
    SONAR IS AN ACRONYM FOR SOUND NAVIGATION
(AND) RANGING.

lens. The blinding by headlights is due to dustlike particles on the posterior surface of the lens acting like ground glass. Typically this will develop first in one eye, or at least be noticed first in one eye. Sometimes patients will not even know they have a cataract in one eye. This is because their other eye may continue to give normal vision for many years.

We all have a dominant eye and a subdominant eye. To figure out which is which in your case, hold your hand out in front of you as if you were shooting a pistol. Close one eye. The eye that is open is your dominant eye. It is the one you use primarily, while the other eye serves to provide stereoscopic, or in-depth, vision.

You might develop a cataract in your subdominant eye and not know it for years. Then you might close your dominant eye for some reason, to rub it, say, and you might notice that the vision in the remaining eye has decreased. This could take place months, even years, after the eye began developing a cataract.

On the other hand, if one develops in your dominant eye, you will notice it much sooner.

If you also had good distance vision but needed glasses for reading, and now you see clearly up close without glasses but have poor distance vision, that is also a sign of cataracts.

Remember: A cataract causes only two symptoms in the beginning of its development: a slight darkening of the image, or a dazzling blindness when bright lights shine into your eye.

Any other symptom is not a cataract and should be looked into immediately.

Such is the case if you see a curtain or wall of blindness coming up from the ground, giving you half your usual field of vision. This is not a cataract but could be a retinal detachment. Check it out with a doctor as quickly as possible. (Chapter 6 will discuss whom you should see about these symptoms.)

Another symptom: If you see a general mistiness or

halos around lights, this is probably not a cataract, but it could be glaucoma. Something else that might be attributed to glaucoma, or a brain condition, is if you can see clearly straight ahead, but on the side you have very little vision. In all these instances, get immediate attention.

Also get to a doctor if you have a sudden loss of vision or a sudden loss of a portion of your field of vision. Again, this is not a cataract, but it could be a retinal detachment or the closing off of an artery—like a stroke in the eye.

Before we go on to the next chapter and cataract surgery, let us quickly review the structure of your eye:

1. The *cornea* is the outer lens that starts the focusing of light.

2. The *aqueous humor* is a fluid rich in vitamin C and other nutrients that bathes the lens.

3. The *iris,* the diaphragm of the eye, controls the amount of light entering the eye.

4. The *lens* itself fine-focuses the light onto the retina.

5. The *zonules,* or ligaments, hold the lens in place.

6. The *vitreous humor* is the clear jelly behind the zonules. It fills most of the eye and stabilizes the retina.

7. The *retina* is the "film" in your "camera."

8. The *sclera,* or white of the eye, is the semirigid structure that surrounds most of the eyeball, except in front of the cornea.

3

Surgery for
Your Cataract

Having a cataract does not mean you have to have surgery.

If you noticed that your vision had decreased, if you had any of the signals we discussed in the last chapter, and if you went to an ophthalmologist who confirmed your suspicion that you had a cataract—THIS IS THE TIME FOR YOU TO STOP AND THINK.

The most important thing for you to know is that allowing a cataract to progress does *not* compromise the final outcome of surgery. This is true in almost every case. We will discuss the few exceptions later on.

But if you have the usual type of cataract, you have a decision to make—and only you can and should make it. That is what I tell patients who come to me and say, "You're the doctor; you tell me when I need the operation." This may be a flattering vote of confidence, but it is not realistic for me—or for any other doctor—to tell anyone what his or her personal needs are.

For example, if you are a brain surgeon, even the slightest trace of cataract requires surgery in order for you to perform your function. If, on the other hand, you are retired and are able to read and take care of your affairs with little or no inconvenience, the surgery should not be performed. Cataracts do not inevitably progress. They can remain stationary for many, many years.

You should also take into consideration the fact that we

no longer have to wait until a cataract is ripe (hardened) to operate. This gives you another option.

Say you have a dense cataract in one eye and a developing one in the other. Then we might wish to operate on the first eye before the second loses its vision.

Again, the basic question you must ask yourself is, "Is my life seriously affected by the amount of vision I have lost?"

Keep questioning yourself in this vein: "What things would I like to do that I cannot do because of my cataract?" If, for example, you wish to drive and you cannot, if you like to read and you cannot, if you feel unsafe walking on the street—then on all accounts surgery is advisable.

However, if occasionally you don't recognize a friend on the street when the light is behind him, but you can read and watch TV, you do not drive, and do not feel you are in any danger of hurting yourself—DON'T GET PUSHED INTO AN OPERATION.

One of the exceptions to this general rule is the rare case of a hypermature cataract. In this type, the lens becomes rapidly clouded and filled with fluid. The entire vision in the eye is lost within days, weeks, or months. In some rarer instances, this type of cataract can rupture inside the eye, causing a great deal of pain. Even if this should occur, surgery sometimes can be very successful.

Another type of cataract, the posterior subcapsular cataract, is not very dense, but seriously affects the patient's vision, especially out in the bright light. When viewed by the ophthalmologist with the slit lamp, this cataract appears as dustlike particles on the posterior surface of the lens.

In these cases, it is easier for the patient to know what is going on than for his physician, because in the darkened examining room the patient's vision may be excellent. But out in the real world, as the patient has discovered, he is seriously handicapped. He cannot function at night when lights are shining in his eye; he cannot walk on the street—cannot lead a normal life. Then the patient does not come in and say he may want an operation; he begs for it. And since we do not have to wait until the cataract is ripe, we can remove it easily, especially with the technique of phacoemulsification. This process will be discussed later in this chapter.

What all this boils down to is that, in almost every case, allowing a cataract to progress will not compromise the final outcome of surgery. So if you are told by an ophthalmologist whom you have never checked out that you have an emergency, if he seems excessively anxious to operate, if he is one of the "newspaper headline surgeons," my advice is to immediately get another opinion.

I repeat, there are *very* few ophthalmologists who would do such an unethical thing. But those few surgeons who use public relations may attract patients who can act irrationally, out of fear of losing their vision.

Anesthesia for Cataract Surgery

Most surgeons have a preference for either general anesthesia or local anesthesia. If your doctor has a preference, it is unwise to try to change what he is used to.

Some surgeons prefer general anesthesia because they like the patient to be totally asleep, and would feel ill at ease otherwise. Others, like myself, find general anesthesia unnecessary for a simple cataract operation. I prefer to have a patient sleepy, but able to respond, under local anesthesia.

If you do have general anesthesia, here is what it is like:

You are given an injection in the vein to put you to sleep. Then after sleep occurs, a tube is passed through your mouth and into your trachea (wind pipe). Through this tube, anesthetic gas will be pumped into your lungs. In essence, the anesthesiologist is "breathing" for you by pumping the gas into your lungs. The gas is mixed with oxygen, and your pulse and blood pressure are closely monitored.

For long operations, general anesthesia is the best solution. But there are some aftereffects. There usually is some nausea and disorientation, and there may be vomiting. The patient must stay in bed for several hours.

With this type of anesthesia the patient knows absolutely nothing about what took place during his surgery. I am not too sure whether this is a great advantage, given the other discomforts. However, this method is recommended for children.

Now for local anesthesia:

The patient receives an injection in the buttocks while still in his room. This makes him slightly drowsy, and by the time he gets to the operating room, he is usually lightly sleeping. When the surgeon touches him on the shoulder, however, he responds.

At that point a very small injection is given in the cheek to deaden sensation around the eye. Then a small injection is given under the lid. By now the patient does not feel anything at all. Usually he is awake and calm, or lightly asleep, depending on the amount of medication given. In most cases the medication is Valium.

Although I use local anesthesia, I have an anesthesiologist standing by, administering the Valium and other sedatives intravenously in case the patient gets restless.

Most of the time, the patient has no recollection of the surgery and feels no pain during the operation or afterward. And, of course, the great advantage of local anesthesia is that when he gets back to his room, the patient can sit up, have a meal, and take a walk. There are none of the other side effects. And so for a cataract operation—which usually takes twenty to forty minutes—I think it is the best way.

Types of Surgery

Now that the anesthetics are out of the way, we can talk about the types of actual surgery.

Let me preface this by saying that there has been a lot of publicity regarding "microsurgery." All this means is that a surgeon is using an operating microscope to enlarge his view of the eye while he is operating. This affords him a more accurate placement of the sutures, the stitches, and the vast majority of surgeons in this country use it today. Any headline heralding *microsurgery—a new technique for cataracts* is a fake.

Types of Cataract Extraction

There are three types of cataract extraction: intracapsular, extracapsular, and phacoemulsification.

Intracapsular Extraction

By now you must realize that I am using big words and giving you a great deal of information so that you will understand the procedures followed and the options available.

So, here is what intracapsular extraction is. Surrounding the mass of the cloudy lens there is a thin layer, similar to plastic wrapping, called the capsule. It is called the anterior capsule in front of the cataract, and the posterior capsule behind the cataract, although the layer is actually continuous and encloses the cataract like the skin of an orange. Since intracapsular means "inside the capsule," it means the cataract is taken out while inside the capsule. In other words, the whole cataract is removed, including the capsule.

To remove the cataract, a semicircular cut is first made halfway around the eye, to allow room for the entire cataract to be removed.

In order to fixate, or grasp, the cataract, freezing is employed. In this technique, a cold probe touches the cataract (see figure 2). When the surgeon lifts on the probe, the cataract is lifted out at the same time (see figure 3).

I introduced this method in the United States in 1962, though credit goes to Dr. Tadeaus Krwawicz, who first used it in Poland. Shortly after I described it at the American Academy of Ophthalmology, most of the other surgeons in the United States adopted the technique.

One advantage of this method is that surgeons have had a high success rate with it.

Another advantage of intracapsular surgery is that when the entire lens, including the capsule, is removed, and when this is successful, there is almost no chance of an after-cataract, or secondary clouding, which would require another operation.

On the other side of the coin, there are disadvantages to intracapsular surgery. One is that, in a small percentage of cases, some of the vitreous jelly can come out of the eye along with the cataract. This leads to a higher incidence of retinal detachment, swelling of the retina, and glaucoma. This happens in well under 5 percent of the cases; even with vitreous loss, however, there is not always an accompanying visual problem.

Another disadvantage of intracapsular surgery is that the incision going halfway around the eye requires anywhere from five to ten stitches (see figure 4, *left*). This necessitates a fairly long period, about one month, during which the patient cannot be active.

Following intracapsular surgery, a lens implant can be used, either attached to the iris or in front of it in the anterior chamber. In most cases, this gives excellent results.

If your surgeon does intracapsular surgery, and can use an implant if you desire it, and if the convalescence time is not important to you, *there is absolutely no reason to switch to another surgeon for another technique.*

Extracapsular Extraction

Now let us examine extracapsular surgery. This is another technique for removal of the cataract through a fairly large incision. It is similar to intracapsular extraction, but leaves the entire posterior capsule or part of it (see figures 5 and 6).

One of the advantages of extracapsular extraction, according to many ophthalmologists, is that leaving the support of the posterior capsule helps prevent retinal detachment and macular edema, or swelling of the retina.

Leaving the posterior capsule also greatly decreases the possibility of vitreous coming out of the eye along with the cataract.

Another advantage is that many surgeons use the posterior capsule as a means of supporting an implant.

In many instances during the surgery, a small hole is

made in the posterior capsule to prevent it from clouding up. This clouding is a disadvantage of extracapsular extraction. Sometimes, if the capsule is left in place, it becomes cloudy and has to be opened later on. Fortunately, a new technique has been developed whereby the capsule can be opened weeks, months, or even years after the surgery, with the use of a special laser, without any hospitalization or cutting.

Indeed, I wrote the first draft of this chapter on an airplane, returning from Paris, where the special laser was developed by Dr. Daniele Aron-Rosa. I had just taken a course in its use.

Thanks to this development, it is now possible to leave the posterior capsule in place in every case, resulting in a healthier eye. Only in those cases where it clouds up will the capsule be opened. This can be done in the doctor's office, with a five-second procedure, using this very special laser.

Another disadvantage of extracapsular extraction is that the surgeon must be specially trained, since it is a somewhat more complicated operation than the intracapsular method. It requires more complex equipment, such as a sophisticated irrigation and aspiration device to wash out the peripheral parts of the cataract. Still another disadvantage is that extracapsular extraction requires a fairly large incision and four to six weeks of relative inactivity afterward. This does not mean staying in bed, or even at home, but there cannot be any heavy lifting, bending, or vigorous physical activity.

Phacoemulsification

The third type of cataract surgery is phacoemulsification, a procedure that I invented in 1967.

Let me preface this explanation by saying that there are a lot of erroneous terms used about my type of surgery, simply because *phacoemulsification* is not the easiest word to remember. When you hear people talking about lasers or laser beams for cataract surgery, most likely they mean phacoemulsification. Yet it has nothing at all to do with lasers! There is no laser operation for cataract removal. Lasers are used for retinal detachments and to open the posterior capsule as mentioned above.

Phacoemulsification is done with an ultrasonic needle that passes into the eye through a relatively small incision (see figure 7). The needle then sucks out the cataract (see figures 8, 9, and 10).

With this technique, the posterior capsule is left intact. This makes it a kind of extracapsular extraction, but the important differences are the use of the high-frequency vibrating needle and the small incision.

The greatest advantage of phacoemulsification is that there is an almost immediate recovery. The next day, all activities are allowed, even a return to work. This is possible because only one suture is placed.

You must be certain before insisting on a phacoemulsification that your surgeon is one with a great deal of practice with that technique. In my opinion, only those who do a lot of surgery—several cases a week—should be performing this operation. The others would be better off doing intracapsular extraction—which, as I said, gives excellent results—or extracapsular extraction.

If you are interested in very rapid rehabilitation, ask your surgeon whether he does phacoemulsification and, if so, how many cases he does a week.

If he says he does not do it, or only does it rarely, ask him to refer you to a surgeon who is highly experienced in the technique, or else *allow him to do the procedure with which he is most familiar.*

Phacoemulsification, in combination with an implant, requires that the incision be opened slightly more to put the implant in. In this case, instead of one stitch, your eye will probably have two or three. But this will usually allow you total freedom of activity within a week.

As I have said, with phacoemulsification the posterior capsule is left in place, either intact, or with a small window in it. It can be used for fixation of the implant, or the implant can be put in front of the iris with equally good results. If the posterior capsule should opacify later, the laser can be used to open it.

What About Outpatient Cataract Surgery?

Throughout the country today we find facilities being opened where cataract surgery is being performed as an outpatient procedure. Instead of staying overnight or longer in a hospital, the patient enters the facility in the morning, has the operation, and leaves several hours later.

Is this the sensible solution for you? The answer depends on various factors. If you have any other kind of medical problem, such as a heart condition, you should not have outpatient cataract surgery. You may need sophisticated support before, during, or after your operation. If you have other serious medical problems, or suspect you do, your place is in the hospital.

On the other hand, if you are in good health and have recently had a checkup, and do not have high blood pressure or diabetes or any bleeding tendency, you might consider such a facility. I believe that phacoemulsification's small incision lends itself to outpatient surgery better than the intracapsular method, where the incision is large. Many qualified ophthalmic surgeons, however, would argue this point with me.

In any case, the general reputation of the facility should be considered, because cleanliness and sterility are vital to any surgery, especially eye surgery.

If it is difficult for you to question patients in the doctor's waiting room because of the in-and-out nature of his practice, remember that it is both ethical and wise for you to ask him for the names of a patient or two who have undergone surgery. Follow up by calling the names he gives you. But keep in mind that he will, naturally, as I would,

tend to give you the names of patients who have had good
results.

Recovery from Surgery

On the day following cataract surgery, if the patient has
had phacoemulsification with a two- or three-millimeter
incision, he is allowed all activities, including most non-
violent sports, and he may return to work. He wears a pair
of sunglasses or his own glasses until he gets his contact
lens or spectacles. This will be discussed in Chapter 8. At
night, even the phacoemulsification patient should wear a
shield over his eye to keep the pillow from pressing on it.

If the patient has an extracapsular or intracapsular extraction, the incision is larger, and although he can walk
around, he should be careful not to indulge in any stren-
uous activities, strain on the toilet, or bend over, as these
increase abdominal pressure and might cause the incision
to rupture. With either of these procedures, physical exer-
cise is forbidden for about a month.

The patient can, in a few days, resume a very moderately
active life-style, and after about a month he can resume all
his normal activities. For many patients, this rehabilitation is not inconvenient at all.

With an implant, the rehabilitation of the patient is not
very different, except that with a phacoemulsification, the
incision must be made slightly larger in order to get the
implant in. Therefore, the patient cannot indulge in heavy
activities on the day following surgery, but must wait a
week or so.

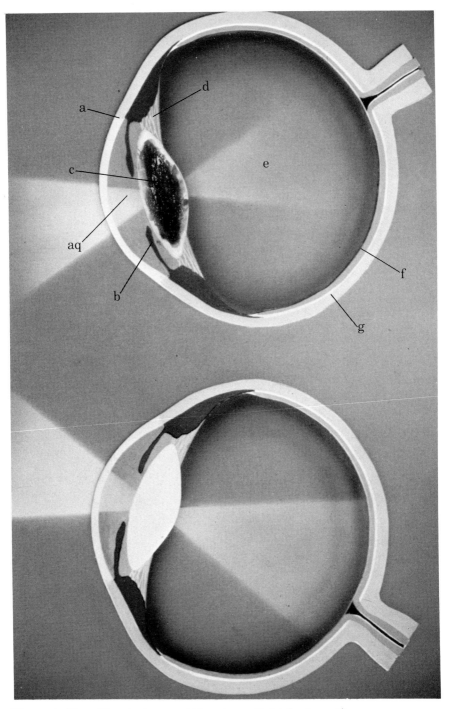

Figure 1. *Top:* Cloudy lens, cutting down light (cataract)
Bottom: Clear lens

a. cornea
b. iris
c. lens (cataract)
d. zonules (ligaments)

e. vitreous humor (jelly)
f. retina
g. sclera
aq. aqueous humor

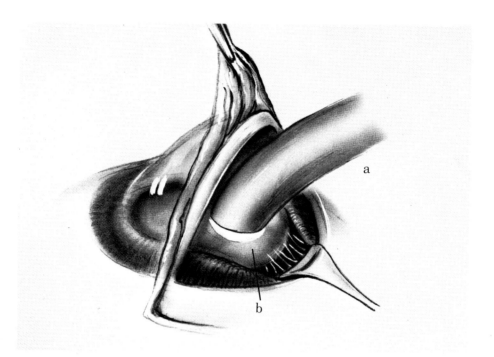

Figure 2. Cryoprobe (a) touching cataract (b)

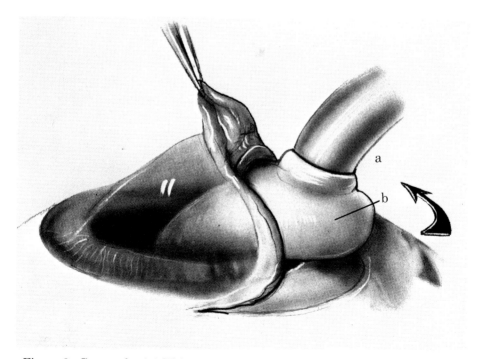

Figure 3. Cryoprobe (a) lifting out cataract (b)

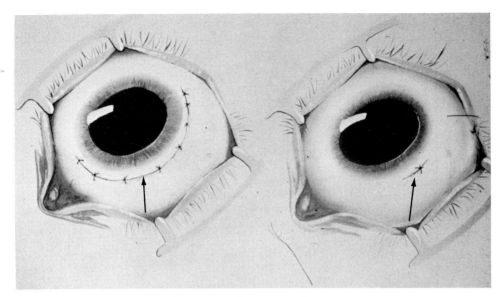

Figure 4. *Left:* Incision for intracapsular cataract surgery
Right: Incision for phacoemulsification cataract surgery

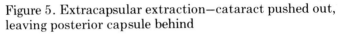

Figure 5. Extracapsular extraction—cataract pushed out,
leaving posterior capsule behind

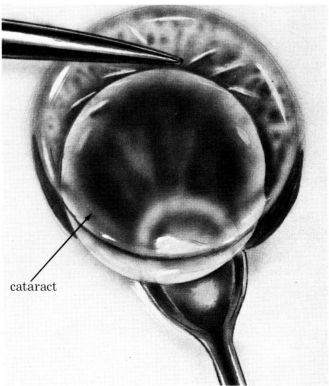

cataract

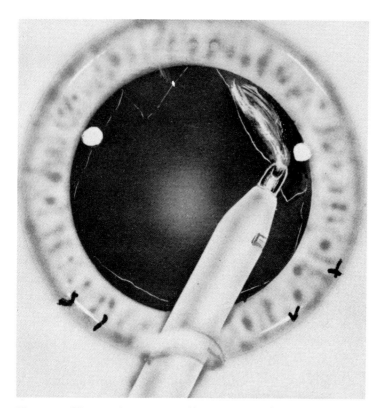

Figure 6. Vacuuming out small remnants of cataract

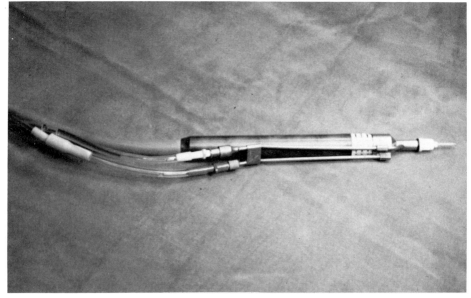

Figure 7. Ultrasonic handpiece and needle

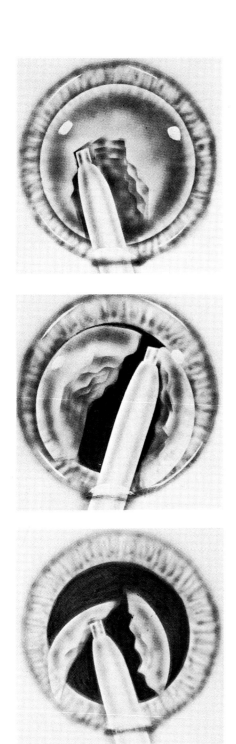

Figures 8, 9, 10.
Ultrasonic needle breaking up and dissolving cataract

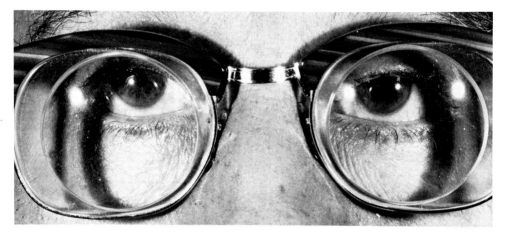

Figure 11. Cataract glasses

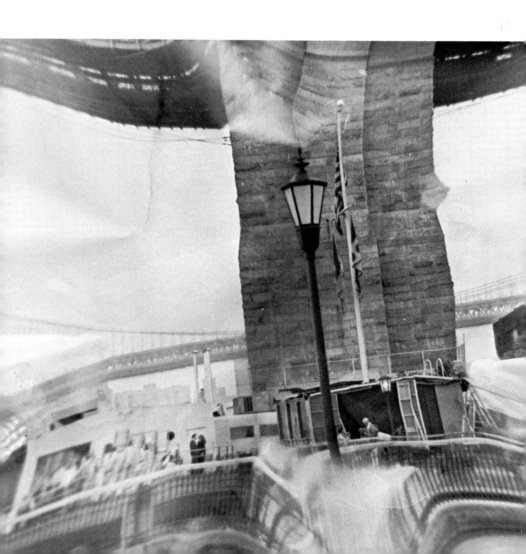

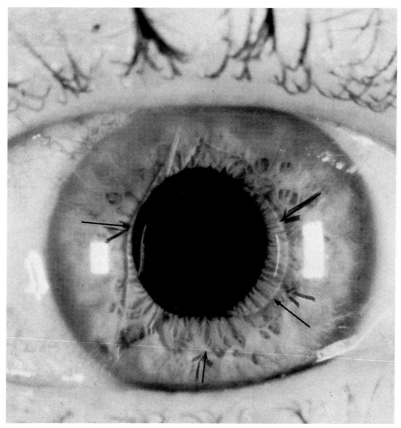

Figure 13. Kelman implant: The tiny man-made lens is *inside* the eye.

Figure 12.
Image as seen with cataract glasses

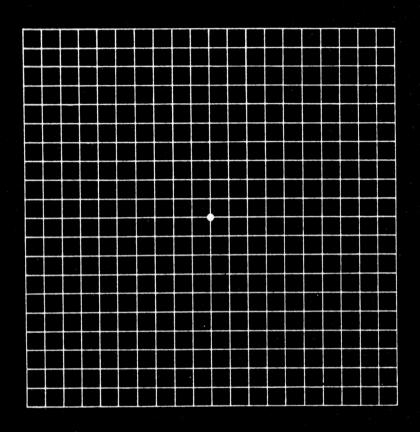

Figure 14. Amsler grid

4

Conditions That Can Complicate Your Surgery

With any of the surgical techniques described in the last chapter, the success rate is well over 95 percent. However, there are a few conditions that do affect the final outcome, and if you have one of these, you may be more prone to complications. These conditions are myopia, glaucoma, diabetes, macular degeneration, bleeding tendencies, and the tendency to poor wound healing.

Myopia

Myopia, or nearsightedness, is the condition wherein the patient, without glasses, can see only if he holds something very close to his eyes. The distant world is extremely blurred. During his school years he had to sit up front, or wear very thick glasses at all times.

One of the effects of this condition is that the eyeball stretches and actually becomes somewhat larger than average. You may not know it, but the tissues of the eye are capable of stretching. The sclera, the outer shell (the white part) of the eye, becomes thin from the stretching but still retains enough strength to support the eyeball.

The blood vessels also stretch, and though they are thinned, they are still able to nourish the structures of the eye. In fact, all the structures stretch harmlessly except the retina, which in many cases becomes extremely thinned and somewhat degenerated.

The danger for this type of patient is that the thinned retina may later detach, especially if the vitreous jelly is lost during the operation. Extracapsular extraction is safer for a case of this sort since the posterior capsule, which prevents the jelly from coming forward, is left wholly or partly intact.

If the retina does not become detached, its thinning can cause a significant decrease in the positive outcome of cataract surgery simply because of the stretching and degeneration.

If you have had a retinal detachment earlier in your life and now need a cataract operation in that same eye, there is an increased chance of the retina's detaching once more. Here again, in my opinion, an extracapsular type of extraction would be safer.

Glaucoma

This condition is one in which the pressure of the eye is consistently too high and the optic nerves are compressed. Glaucoma is usually painless, but it affects the peripheral vision, at times leaving the person with only a central island of sight. Sometimes the person is totally unaware of this gradual loss. What usually makes cataract surgery for a glaucoma sufferer more difficult is that such a person's pupils are usually constricted (made smaller) by eye drops to control the pressure. In order for the surgeon to do a cataract operation, it is necessary to dilate, or enlarge, the pupil. Very often, years of using constricting drops cannot be overcome at the time of surgery. The surgeon is then faced with an operation through a very tiny pupil, and this can sometimes lead to complications.

If you have long-standing glaucoma and have been using drops for many years, ask your surgeon if he has had adequate experience with this type of case (most surgeons have). If not, ask him to refer you to a glaucoma-cataract specialist. Interestingly enough, after a successful cataract operation, pressures in the eye from the glaucoma frequently normalize. This is because the drainage areas for the fluid are now somewhat opened up.

Diabetes

Diabetes that develops later in life, in the middle fifties, usually has very little effect on the eye. This is often the type of diabetes that can easily be controlled with diet or minimal medication, and it usually does not compromise the results of cataract surgery.

The type of diabetes that often affects the outcome of cataract surgery is the diabetes that has developed from the time of the patient's adolescence or early adult years. After fifteen to twenty years from the onset of diabetes, a degeneration appears in the retina, *whether or not medication is taken for it*. This degeneration is called diabetic retinopathy, and it consists of hemorrhages and fluid leaks in the nerve areas of the retina. This considerably reduces vision. I repeat, *these changes do not come about until the patient has had controlled or uncontrolled diabetes for fifteen to twenty years.*

If you have had diabetes for that many years and are now faced with a cataract operation, you can probably expect that your vision will not be 20/20 following the surgery, but that there will be a reduction in your central vision. In some cases, this condition can be arrested with the use of a laser, and if this is so in your condition, your ophthalmologist will certainly recommend this treatment for you.

Macular Degeneration

This is the condition referred to by your doctor when he says you have hardening of the arteries in the back of your eye. We do not really know the cause of this condition, but it is a localized degeneration at the macula, the most sensitive portion of the retina, involving your central vision.

Macular degeneration, like diabetes (that is, long-standing diabetes), can significantly affect the outcome of your surgery, leaving you with little or no central vision or ability to read print. This can happen even though the surgery was perfectly performed. Macular degeneration is something that usually happens at the age of seventy and upward, but occasionally it can be seen in younger patients.

It is sometimes impossible for the surgeon to diagnose macular degeneration prior to the surgery. In fact, it is one of the leading causes of disappointment on a patient's part following technically successful cataract surgery.

Bleeding Tendencies

There are other, less common, causes of problems in surgery, such as bleeding tendencies, which can cause a hemorrhage during and after the operation.

Poor Wound Healing

Another problem is the tendency to poor wound healing. However, this and the tendency to bleed are rare and can easily be controlled in most cases with proper medication.

5

The Operation: What You Experience

While the actual details of the operation may vary from surgeon to surgeon and from patient to patient, the overall series of events in a cataract operation are more or less standard throughout the United States. A description of a cataract operation as performed by me in New York, therefore, will give you a pretty good idea of what to expect.

Before going to the hospital, the patient is instructed to have a physical examination conducted by his own physician. Although being admitted to the hospital is not a terribly traumatic procedure, it is still an event of some consequence in a person's life. If the patient has some predisposing condition requiring treatment before admission to the hospital, the patient's own doctor would be able to diagnose such a condition and adequately treat it. This would spare the patient an unnecessary admission to the hospital followed by an immediate discharge if he was not physically able to have surgery. This explains why a patient should be examined by his own physician first.

Once in the hospital, however, it is important that the patient be examined again on the day before surgery to make sure nothing new has cropped up since the patient was examined by his own doctor and also to make certain again for everybody's protection that the outside doctor did not overlook any condition that could be of importance in the patient's surgery or recuperation. In most cases the second examination turns up nothing new. In the very few cases where something important is picked up in the hospital, however, it is well worth the extra time and effort.

So when the patient arrives at the hospital, the day prior to surgery, he goes to the admitting office of the hospital where various insurance forms and other clerical tasks are completed. From here the patient is admitted to a room where he can relax for a few minutes until some laboratory tests are performed. These tests, which include a urinalysis, a chest X ray, and a blood analysis, are done for the protection of the patient, the hospital, and the doctor. They are to ascertain whether the patient has diabetes, any bleeding tendency, hypertension, kidney disease, or any other condition that could compromise the outcome of the surgery. Then a physical examination is conducted by the hospital's staff doctor or internist for the very same reasons.

A sixty-four-year-old patient was examined the last week in November by his internist and found to be in good health. In the middle of December, when the patient arrived at the hospital, he said he felt fine but he had had what he termed a period of indigestion. When an electrocardiogram was run in the hospital, it was discovered that the patient had had a very recent although mild heart attack. The cataract surgery was then postponed and the patient was treated as a heart patient until he was out of danger. If the in-hospital examination had not been made, the patient might never have known that he had a heart attack until much later, when a second heart attack could have been more serious.

Once the tests are finished, the patient can relax for the rest of the day and exchange stories with the other patients who are there for the same reason. In my practice, five or six patients are operated on the same day. Usually in this group there is at least one patient who has already had cataract surgery in the first eye and this patient becomes the group leader and answers any remaining questions that the other patients may have. Because the patients in my practice are brought to the hospital together, stay on the same floor, and are driven back to the office together, many of them become good friends. In one case, two patients who shared their cataract experience eventually got married! Naturally, I cannot promise you that result with every cataract operation.

That evening after a light dinner the patient is given a sedative and generally is able to sleep soundly until morning.

In the morning a nurse comes to the room and gives the patient an injection in the buttocks, which relaxes the patient and makes him slightly drowsy. This injection does not put the patient to sleep; it is simply a tranquilizer. The nurse also puts drops into the patient's eye (which is usually marked by an X to make certain that the correct eye is treated), and more drops are put in over the next hour or so, until the pupil is well dilated for surgery.

Finally someone comes with a trolley (a stretcher on wheels), and the patient is wheeled to the operating room. Here the doctor greets the patient, takes a look at the eye, and massages it gently with his fingers or places some type of weighted bag on it to soften it. An injection is now given at the side to the patient's face; the patient usually only feels the first pinprick as the needle goes in, since the anesthetic solution takes effect immediately.

Next the operating-room nurse disinfects the eye with various solutions and flushes it out with sterile salt water. None of this is uncomfortable and generally the nurses try to make the patient feel at ease. Just before beginning the operation, the surgeon gives the patient one final injection near the eye to prevent the eye from moving and the lid from closing during the operation. This injection also is painless in almost every case and works in a few seconds.

The patient is then draped, or covered with sterile cloths. Although the nose and mouth may be lightly covered by the drapes, there is always plenty of air for the patient to breathe. In my practice, we have an anesthesiologist standing by with an intravenous drip going so that should the patient need additional sedation, it can be given without further injection.

The patient is awake and can converse with the surgeon, which is of great value to the patient's peace of mind. You have no doubt who is doing your surgery, since you can speak with the doctor who is operating directly over your head. Because of some published stories, many patients wonder whether their doctor or some other doctor did the operation. I can assure you that the cases of "ghost surgery" in the private practice of medicine are today very few and far between.

During the operation the patient may hear the surgeon talking to the nurse or to other doctors who may be observing. He may hear the noises of the various instruments or the buzzing of the phacoemulsifier, but none of these is terrifying in any way. The operation is bloodless, and in most cases is extremely easy for the accomplished surgeon.

Anytime from fifteen to forty minutes later, the operation is over, and the patient is returned to his room after a brief stay in the recovery room.

By this time the tranquilizer has pretty much worn off and the patient can safely sit up, walk around, and eat a meal. There is generally no pain and no discomfort. Most patients are amazed at how easy the whole experience is, although naturally they are all glad when it is over.

During that day and night the patient may receive eye drops from the nurse. The next morning, after the eye is examined, the patient is discharged. This is modern cataract surgery as practiced by many ophthalmologists throughout the United States today.

6

The Postoperative Period

In the postoperative period, following cataract surgery, you should be aware of the symptoms that are normal and those that are not. The symptoms are basically the same with all the different types of cataract surgery, except that they will be more marked with the large-incision intracapsular and extracapsular types than they will be for phacoemulsification, where the incision is only an eighth of an inch long.

Foreign-Body Sensation

The most common unimportant symptom is the sensation of a slight foreign body in the eye. This is due to the one or more sutures, or stitches, and will usually depend in severity on the number of them, their type, and whether the doctor has cut the knots very short. A slight feeling of a cinder in the eye is normal.

An extremely irritating foreign-body sensation that persists more than a few hours is a sign that something is amiss—a suture has opened or was not properly trimmed. It could also be a sign that the cornea is damaged, and if the symptom persists for more than a day, you should call it to the attention of your ophthalmologist. While you are waiting, a very gentle pressure, such as you might get by covering the eye with a few cotton balls held in place by one or two pieces of Scotch tape, should decrease the severity of the symptom.

Tearing (Weeping)

In association with the foreign-body sensation, the eyes often give off some fluid. Here again it is a question of degree. A very slight amount of tearing is normal. But large amounts of fluid running out of the eye suggest an extreme irritation or possibly even a wound leak.

The fluid produced inside the eye is clear, and if one of the sutures has opened and fluid is leaking from the eye, the patient will see this as increased tearing. Fluid running copiously from the eye for more than a few hours is a sign to call your ophthalmologist. If the fluid is pink or blood-tinged or yellow, it is even more important. With phacoemulsification, because the incision is so small, this complication is almost nonexistent.

Photophobia

Again it is a question of degree. A slight discomfort when looking at the bright sky is to be expected. A severe pain in bright areas is a sign that the eye is not properly medicated or that something is wrong. Generally, the patient is most comfortable immediately following surgery with either a light patch on the eye or sunglasses. In my practice, we do not use a patch following surgery, but place a small strainer over the eye, so the patient can see through it and yet be protected. This is for a period of one day, after which sunglasses can be worn.

Floating Silver Dollars

If the surgeon puts air into the anterior chamber (as I do) at the end of the procedure to push the jelly (vitreous) back, this air will slowly be absorbed over the next day or so. In the meantime, the patient will see what looks like floating silver dollars inside his eye. This will last for a day or two, three at the most. Provided that these areas of blackness move about, there is no cause for alarm.

If there is an area of blackness that does *not* move, but remains fixed in your field of vision no matter how much you move your head, this is possibly a cause for alarm since it might be a retinal detachment. Only one in one hundred patients develops retinal detachment, on average. This subject will be discussed later in the chapter.

Complications That Can Occur

Certain complications are common to all types of cataract surgery, but the chance of their occurring varies according to which operation is used. Today, many surgeons are moving toward the extracapsular type of extraction because they feel that it reduces the incidence of such complications as retinal detachment, infection, and swelling of the macula.

I believe that this trend as well as that toward phacoemulsification—which is a type of extracapsular extraction with the additional benefit of the small incision—will be beneficial to more patients in the long run. I should add, however, that those doctors who consider intracapsular extraction to be just as good are recommending it on the basis of their own experience and the excellent results they have obtained with it. So there is absolutely no reason to abandon your surgeon if he tells you that he practices intracapsular extraction. If he was not getting the results he wanted, he would naturally change to another technique.

Infection

The rate of serious infection following cataract surgery varies slightly, from reports around the country, but the accepted average is one in one thousand.

An infection does not mean a slightly red eye with tearing; it means extreme pain, extreme sensitivity to light, and swollen and engorged lids. The pain travels to the top of the patient's head, and feels like a toothache rather than a scratching type of pain from sutures.

Occasionally there is fever, and in many instances the patient feels acutely ill. This rare condition is the most extreme emergency that can follow cataract surgery, and a delay of hours or even minutes in getting treatment can make the difference between getting back some useful vision in the eye or losing the eye completely.

Indeed, the biggest disaster following this type of infection is total loss of the eye, where the eye itself has to be removed. Fortunately, with modern treatment methods, this extremely unfortunate outcome is rarely seen. Serious infection does, however, usually significantly reduce the patient's ability to see.

What causes the infection is germs introduced at the time of surgery, either from the "sterile field"—from the prepared upper half of the patient's face—or from some contamination source in the operating room, and which begin to multiply inside the eye. (Germs can also get in later, from the patient's own hands or from contaminated medication.)

A few germs can easily be taken care of by the body's natural defenses. If this were not so, almost every eye would become infected, because even in the most sterile of sterile fields, there are germs. Sometimes, a germ entering the eye is so virulent that it can overcome the body's defense mechanism. When these bacteria begin to multiply they do so at a frenzied rate.

One of the most feared germs in the eye is pyocyaneus, a rare germ that can destroy the eye in a matter of hours. Usually, though, the germ is not that powerful, and it would take several days to destroy the eye if left unattended.

Immediate hospitalization, with antibiotics given intravenously as well as orally and injections of antibiotics around the eye and, in some cases, cortisone, can in many instances save the sight of the eye. Sometimes a second operation called a vitrectomy can be used to prevent the progression of the infection toward the retina. In a vitrectomy, the vitreous jelly is removed with a surgical instrument so that the bacteria that are working their way back toward the retina can be removed before they can do damage.

To make the diagnosis in which germs are involved, the surgeon will place a very tiny needle in the anterior chamber of the eye and draw out a small amount of fluid for culture. He will then give the patient antibiotics while the culture is growing, and in two days or sooner he will have his results. These tell him whether the antibiotics he was using are the correct ones. If not, he can change course and give an antibiotic specific to the germ in the patient's eye.

This is one of the reasons surgeons do not operate on both eyes at the same time. Although the odds of getting an infection in both eyes would be even smaller than one in a thousand, the chance still exists. The ultimate catastrophe of two infected eyes, no matter how infinitesimal the risk, is an unacceptable one.

So, if you feel a tremendous pain and a change in your vision, with swollen lids and even a slight fever—or maybe even no fever—it is time to make an emergency visit immediately to your doctor or to an eye hospital. Infection can occur anytime from hours following the surgery to weeks or months later. If it occurs several months after the operation, instead of a bacterial infection it is usually a fungus one, which can also be treated with the proper antibiotics.

Corneal Edema

The cornea, the watch-glass crystal of the eye, is maintained in its transparent state by a delicate layer of cells on the inner surface. These cells pump fluid out of the cornea, thereby maintaining its clarity. When these cells are diseased or damaged, the cornea becomes cloudy.

If the patient has a diseased cellular layer (a condition called endothelial dystrophy), sometimes the eye will not tolerate cataract surgery. This is impossible to predict absolutely before surgery, but frequently a cell count can alert the surgeon to possible dangers. In any case, damaging these delicate cells can cause a thickening and whitening of the cornea, reducing the patient's vision postoperatively. Fortunately, this only lasts about two to three weeks in most cases. In less than half of 1 percent of the cases it lasts longer.

If the cornea does not clear up after several months of treatment, a corneal graft could be necessary. This requires taking the corneal donor "button" from someone recently deceased, removing a button from the patient's eye, and replacing it with the donor button. Happily, this is an operative procedure with a high rate of success.

Corneal edema can also come postoperatively from high pressure in the eyes (glaucoma).

Glaucoma

Usually, preexisting glaucoma conditions are improved following cataract surgery, but in rare cases they get worse. The patient notices a haziness in his vision, and the doctor records a high pressure in the eye. Fortunately, this condition is usually amenable to medical therapy, and only rarely is surgery required.

Macular Edema

In the very center of the retina where the most important vision, the reading vision, is located, is an area called the macula. For reasons still unknown to us, sometimes after perfect surgery—in about 20 percent of all cases—the macula becomes swollen some time afterward, even up to two years later, and the patient's vision drops dramatically. This is usually no cause for alarm, and simply requires patience, because in almost every case the vision does eventually return, usually within weeks, but sometimes taking a year to do so. In only a few instances is the vision permanently impaired. Cortisone is sometimes helpful for this condition, as are other anti-inflammatory agents.

If following cataract surgery you have seen very well and suddenly your central vision drops, chances are you have macular edema. This is easily diagnosed in the doctor's office with a fluorescein angiogram, which is a picture of your retina, taken after a dye has been injected in the vein of your arm.

If the macula is swollen, the dye leaks out of it and shows up in the photograph. It does not indicate a poor operation, or any surgical mishap. It can occur after the most perfect surgery.

Retinal Detachment

The retina, you will remember, is like the film in a camera, and is attached to the inner surface of the hard shell of the eye, the sclera. Even without cataract surgery, the retina can detach, but after cataract surgery, even perfect surgery, anywhere from 1 to 2 percent of patients do have a retinal detachment. If you are very nearsighted, your chances of retinal detachment are somewhat higher, perhaps 4 to 5 percent.

The symptom of a retinal detachment is what looks like a curtain, or a wall, usually black in color, coming up from the ground. Or, more rarely, it seems to be coming down toward the ground. (Only blackness is seen on the wall itself.) This is cause for an immediate visit to the ophthalmologist, and if a retinal detachment is diagnosed, hospitalization very soon thereafter is usually advisable.

If the condition is detected early enough, in many cases the retina can be reattached surgically, with little loss in vision. About 15 percent of retinal detachments, however, are not reparable and lead to a permanent loss of vision. Again, retinal detachment can occur after the most perfect surgery.

Sometimes a special ophthalmologist, a retinologist, is called in to do this somewhat specialized reattachment surgery, but many ophthalmologists are able to do the procedure themselves.

Hemorrhage

The blood vessels of the eye are delicate, and especially in a predisposed patient—that is, one with diabetes or heart disease—the blood vessels can break.

Also, in order to heal, the incision must have blood vessels grow across it. If a patient exerts himself unduly, these blood vessels can rupture and bleed into the eye. Obviously, the larger the incision, the more this is apt to happen. So here again, the smaller incision of phacoemulsification is an advantage, especially for those patients who must be active fairly soon after their operation.

A small hemorrhage will rapidly darken the vision, and may even eliminate it, but there is not a clearly defined wall, as in retinal detachment. In any case, it is an emergency, and you should see your ophthalmologist right away. Because the bleeding is very often associated with a rise in pressure inside the eye, it must be treated medically.

A small hemorrhage in the front of the eye, in the anterior chamber, usually clears with no problems. A hemorrhage in the vitreous will also clear, but it sometimes requires several months to do so.

The worst type of hemorrhage is the one called an expulsive hemorrhage, which occurs in very, very rare cases on the operating table, usually with total loss of sight. In this most unfortunate occurrence, during the surgery the eye begins to bleed, pushing off the retina and destroying any chance for subsequent vision. The incidence of this is less than one in five thousand cases.

Retained Lens Material

Sometimes, in a cataract extraction, some cataract particles are not visible to the surgeon at the time of surgery and are left inside the eye. If these remnants are from the soft, outer part of the cataract (cortex), they will usually be absorbed in some weeks or several months. During this time, however, the vision may be reduced.

It the remnants are from the harder central portion (nucleus), they may have to be removed surgically if the eye is inflamed. Fortunately this complication is rare and is usually associated with extracapsular surgery, but can also be seen with intracapsular surgery if the capsule breaks during the cataract extraction.

Other Reasons for Imperfect Vision After Surgery

As I said before, removal of a cataract, even perfectly, does not guarantee perfect vision. Perfect vision depends not only on a clear lens (absence of a cataract) but also on proper functioning of the other structures of the eye. In some cases, removal of the cataract still leaves the eye with other problems that were present before.

When a cataract is very dense, the surgeon may often be unable to diagnose these preexisting problems before the operation. Just as the patient cannot see out of the eye, the surgeon cannot see into it.

This is one of the most frustrating things for both the doctor and the patient. It also is the leading cause of dissatisfaction on the part of patients. Picture this situation: The ophthalmologist sees a patient with a cataract and tells him that most likely after its removal he will see well. The operation goes well, the eye heals, but postoperatively the patient's vision is poor. Naturally the patient assumes that the doctor did something wrong; the operation was "botched."

Not so. Following are some of the conditions, other than cataracts, that can preexist and reduce the final vision.

Amblyopia

This is frequently called a lazy eye. As the name implies, that particular eye did not learn to see well when the patient was a child, probably because the eye turned in or out. Since the eye was not properly used from the start, the vision in it never developed to its maximum. If later in life such an eye develops a cataract and the cataract is removed, the postoperative vision will not be 20/20. It will only return to the best vision that the patient had, at the age of nine or ten years. Very often, if it is a severely amblyopic eye, that vision is very poor.

Sometimes the patient is unaware that he had an amblyopic eye. Similarly, if the cataract is dense, the condition cannot be diagnosed by the physician, especially with small degrees of amblyopia.

Additionally frustrating is the fact that there is no known treatment for this condition.

Senile Macular Degeneration

In order to help the patient understand this condition, the ophthalmologist will often describe it as "hardening of the arteries of the back of the eye," a condition to which it is similar.

Once a person passes the age of sixty, the macula—the highly sensitive and critical area of the eye that you use for reading—can become dried out or hardened or degenerated and the nerves in that area will die. This condition is localized and confined to the central reading vision area, and it does not lead to blindness of the entire eye.

There is no cure for this degeneration. The disappointment and unhappiness it causes are all too familiar to ophthalmologists, and the man who discovers the treatment for this disease, or its prevention, deserves the Nobel Prize, in my opinion.

As to how the condition affects cataract surgery, here again the patient comes in with a dense cataract and the surgeon cannot look into the retina. If it is a "youngish" patient, in his early sixties, the surgeon may confidently tell the patient that he will remove the cataract to restore good vision.

The operation proceeds smoothly, and postoperatively the eye is healing. Then the surgeon suggests a vision test, and the patient's vision turns out to be 20/100, or very poor. The doctor is disappointed that he could not help the patient, and the patient is distraught and angry at the doctor.

This phenomenon occurs in about 7 to 15 percent of elderly patients, and as you can understand, it severely limits the visual results after cataract surgery.

Incidentally, let me explain the notation of 20/100. Both the number 20 and the number 100 refer to feet. Vision of

20/20 means that at 20 feet, a person can read what the average eye can read at 20 feet. So 20/100 means that at 20 feet you can read what the average person can read at 100 feet. In other words, you must get five times closer to an object in order to see it.

Capsular Haze

In extracapsular extraction or phacoemulsification, if the patient has a predisposition to retinal detachment—that is, if he is highly nearsighted and has already had a detachment in either eye—the posterior capsule is often left intact. Remember, this capsule is the back, Saran-Wraplike layer of the cataract. It is usually clear, or can be cleaned at the time of surgery.

When left intact, the capsule holds the vitreous jelly back to support the retina and helps prevent detachment, in the opinion of many surgeons. The problem with leaving it intact is that sometimes, anywhere from two months to two years or even later, it can cloud up. Then the patient, whose vision has been perfect postoperatively, finds it becoming clouded just as it was during the cataract period.

Fortunately, opening the capsule is a very simple procedure, done sterilely and painlessly with a very tiny needle that enters the eye and makes a tiny window in the capsule. Although this is usually done in a surgical suite in the doctor's office or in a hospital, it does not require any postoperative convalescence, and the patient usually can return to his normal activities with perfectly restored vision.

As I mentioned earlier, there is now a laser available to open the posterior capsule nonsurgically if it should cloud up. This procedure is called a Yag laser capsulotomy, and I believe this is going to induce many surgeons to leave the capsule intact in almost every case, since it does provide for a healthier eye.

Diabetic Retinopathy

People who have had diabetes for more than fifteen or twenty years very often develop abnormalities in their retinas, usually, unfortunately, in the central reading area. These abnormalities are in the form of small hemorrhages or loops of blood vessels.

Sometimes this condition can be arrested with another type of laser that has been in use for many years in this country. If you have had long-standing diabetes, a frequent retinal examination—at least once a year—is a good idea.

In the case of a patient who has had diabetes for many years and who has a dense cataract, the surgeon will usually advise that the postoperative vision may or may not be affected by the diabetes. Diabetic hemorrhages, if left untreated, can lead to severe loss of vision.

Hypertensive Retinopathy

In a patient with long-standing and usual high blood pressure, changes somewhat similar to those caused by diabetes are seen in the back of the eye, in the retina. These changes also can lead to disappointment with vision after cataract surgery.

For purposes of this discussion, retinal changes due to high blood pressure can be considered similar to those caused by diabetes. They are sometimes amenable to laser treatment. In any case, a patient with high blood pressure should be checked regularly by his medical doctor, and have the blood pressure brought under control. This will sometimes ameliorate the retinal condition.

These conditions have been listed simply to advise you that they exist. They are, however, relatively rare, and the record of improved sight after cataract surgery is better than 95 percent.

Indeed, ninety-five out of every one hundred patients get a significant improvement in their vision after cataract surgery, and more than seven out of ten usually achieve 20/20 vision.

As I have said, the ability to accomplish this is in the hands of your local ophthalmologist, who has been trained in surgical techniques. You do not have to go to some faraway place to get these excellent results.

Lid Droop

Occasionally after cataract surgery—as after glaucoma surgery or corneal transplant surgery—the lid of the operated eye will be lower than it was before, making the operated eye appear smaller than the other eye. This condition can last up to a year or more. Usually the eye returns to its normal appearance within a month or so. The cause of the condition is not entirely known and it happens in patients who had local and in those who had general anesthesia. The person who is most conscious of this slight lid droop is the patient himself when he looks in the mirror. Other people generally do not notice it at all.

7

Eye Drops and Tests: Why Are They Necessary?

Before and after cataract surgery, your ophthalmologist is likely to use several different drops to help prepare your eye for surgery and aid in its healing after the operation. You can expect to use the drops for a few weeks afterward. I will try to describe the commonly used medications and their effects on your eye and your body.

Some surgeons ask their patients to use eye drops at home for a few days before the operation. These are usually antibiotic drops (most antibiotic eye drops have bottles with white tops). The drops help clean the outside coverings of the eye in preparation for the procedure. Although commonly used, they are not necessary for all cases of surgery. Frequently they are started on the day prior to the operation.

A few hours before your operation is scheduled, your surgeon will probably have ordered a significant amount of eye drops to be used. These include drops to modify the position of your pupil, to allow the cataract to be removed easily. These drops are given at frequent intervals to maximize their effect. Additionally, pills and/or intravenous solutions may be used to help control the pressure inside your eye at the start of the surgery. These medications are used in addition to whatever injections your surgeon may feel will help you be relaxed for your operation.

After the operation, and depending on the type of surgery you have had, eye drops and possibly pills will be used for a few weeks. I shall describe briefly the classes of eye drops employed and how they can be easily recognized by both physician and patient.

Drops that come in containers with red tops are those that dilate the pupil (make it larger). These drops are used several times each day to make the pupil move so that it heals in the proper position. They also tend to relax the muscle inside the eye and give the patient comfort during the healing period. The different types of red-top drops differ mainly in their length of action, and thus the surgeon can completely control how far and how fast the pupil moves each day. He makes his choice based on the type of surgery the patient has had and the progress the patient is making. These drops can be modified at each postoperative visit if necessary.

Drops that come in containers with white tops are generally those that either prevent infection (antibiotics) or control the amount of inflammation and wound healing (steroids). These drops may be in combination form, with antibiotics and steroid preparations mixed together for the sake of convenience. They are also used several times each day during the initial period after surgery and, again, can be adjusted to fit the individual patient's need. They allow for comfort and proper healing of the eye while preventing infection and other problems.

Pills are frequently used in the immediate postoperative period. Diamox® (a white pill the size of an aspirin tablet) can be given to control the amount of fluid produced by the eye and thus help to control the pressure inside the eye. This pill is usually used for a few days after surgery and is then discontinued.

Less commonly, drops in containers with green tops are prescribed. These also change the size of the pupil, but by making the pupil smaller. With certain types of intraocular lens implants, these drops are needed to help position the implant. In some cases, the drops can be used to modify the pressure in the eye or to control the way the pupil heals. Using this type of drop does not mean there is a problem;

rather, your ophthalmologist has different requirements for healing.

Another type of medication that is sometimes used after surgery is cortisone (steroid is another name). This medication is given by mouth and affects the healing process in the eye as well as in the rest of the body. When drops alone are not sufficient to aid in the eye's proper healing, ophthalmologists will prescribe cortisone pills to control the postoperative course.

In most cases, patients having cataract surgery with or without implants have their medicines completely stopped within the first two months after their surgery. It is possible that some drops will be needed on a long-term basis to control the eye more completely. These are generally given just once or twice a day and have very little in the way of adverse reactions.

Any medication can have an undesirable side effect. It is fortunate that eye medicines usually have no untoward effects other than the minor inconvenience of putting in eye drops. Since eye drops and tears drain through a sophisticated mechanism built into your eyelids and nose and wind up in the back of the throat, these drops may be "tasted" after their use. Patients often notice this when they start the drops but usually forget about it after a few days. On rare occasions, allergies to drops exist and manifest themselves as an uncomfortable itching and burning of the eyelids and cheek skin for a matter of hours after the drops are used. More commonly, patients notice a slight stinging or burning which disappears a few minutes after the drops have been placed. This is especially noticed with drops in containers with red tops and is normal.

Drops in containers with green tops give the feeling of a brow ache or forehead headache immediately after their use. Generally this is a temporary feeling and goes away within a few days after the start of the use of these drops.

Diamox, the pill that controls fluid production inside the eye, frequently has some bodily sensations associated with its use. It is common for patients to notice a numbness or tingling in their fingers and toes. Sometimes there is a decrease in appetite and a feeling of stomach upset, as well as a general feeling of being tired. Fortunately all these complaints tend to disappear as soon as the drug is discontinued, usually within the first few days after surgery.

Patients are frequently confused by the order in which to administer their drops, or how much time to allow between drops. The order of drops usually does not matter; if the individual physician feels it is important, he will direct the patient specifically as to this matter.

As for timing, eye drops should not be applied a matter of seconds apart. The result would be to wash one drop out while instilling the other. Instead, let a few minutes (two to five) elapse between instilling the first drop and the second, between the second and the third, and so on. This allows for adequate absorption of each individual medication.

When drops or any other medication is prescribed to be used three or four times a day, it is best to divide the dosages more or less equally throughout the day. This would mean that a three-times-a-day medication would be taken approximately every eight hours. A medication prescribed on a four-times-a-day basis can conveniently be taken at breakfast, lunch, dinner, and bedtime. If more frequent administration is required, the doctor should instruct the patient as to what schedule to use. Full information about how any medicine should be taken is always typed on the prescription label prepared by the pharmacy. The pharmacist will have interpreted the prescription that the physician has written, and will describe in clear, easy-to-read language how the patient should take his medicine. Except in special cases, the name of each medication should be listed on the label of the medication itself. It is useful for the patient to know the name of each medicine he is taking and to have it available when he sees his ophthalmologist. Many patients prefer to actually carry the medicine containers with them to the eye doctor's office, so that the doctor can immediately tell the patient which medicines should be decreased and which may be stopped completely at the time of the patient's visit.

Some patients will be using eye drops even before they

consider having cataract extraction. For example, patients with glaucoma use eye drops daily. These drops should be modified as the ophthalmologist directs. They may or may not be needed again after the operation.

Your doctor and his staff should be ready and anxious to answer all your questions about your eye medications, and you should be able to understand their use and method of administration. Being able to use eye drops implies that the patient knows how to get his drops into his eyes. If this is difficult for you, ask your doctor. He will be happy to show you the proper method of instilling your drops.

Why Do I Need Those Tests?

Certain tests are performed to help your surgeon give you the best treatment. These are the most common ones.

Visual Field Test

This test is performed in a room with low-level lighting and requires the patient to indicate his awareness of a small light or similar target that is moved about on a screen. The purpose of the test is to determine how extensive an area the patient can see when he fixes his gaze at some central point. Typically this test determines the limits of a person's peripheral field of view. It is a subjective test that requires good patient cooperation. This test is often used to evaluate any damage to the retina that may be caused by glaucoma and other eye disorders. If the eye being tested has an advanced cataract, the test may be simplified by the use of a flashlight used as a target. Although this method is limited, it can give some basic information about retinal function.

Tonometry and Tonography

Tonometry measures the pressure of the eye. Excessively high pressure can damage an eye in a matter of hours. Even elevated pressure, over a period of time (such as with un-treated glaucoma) may result in slow, progressive damage to the retina and the peripheral field of view. There are a number of ways of measuring the eye pressure, including an "air puff" device that can measure the pressure without actually touching the eye. The pressure of the eye is an important piece of information for the eye doctor and it is typical that the pressure be measured at each eye examination.

Tonography also measures the eye's pressure but does so under varying conditions and for an extended period of time. A tonograph gives the doctor a chart or graph from which he can extract more information about the eye's pressure and outflow of aqueous.

Endothelial Cell Counting

The endothelial cell layer of the cornea of the eye is involved in keeping the cornea clear and healthy. These cells act as pumping mechanisms, and, should any of them die, they are not replaced. Although normal aging causes a decrease in the number of living cells, eye surgery may cause additional cell loss. For this reason, a count of these cells may be requested by the ophthalmologist so as to be able to determine corneal health. This may be done both preoperatively and postoperatively. A specialized microscope is used to see these cells and photograph them or record them on videotape for later inspection by the doctor. Patients who are possible candidates for an implant lens often undergo this test.

Pachometry

This test measures the thickness of the patient's cornea. The test may be used to help determine corneal health. Pachometry readings may be taken frequently if the corneal shape is believed to be undergoing changes. Pachometry readings are often used when a corneal transplant is being considered.

A Scan

The ophthalmologist uses the A scanner to determine the length of the eyeball so that the proper power of an implant lens may be determined with the help of a computer.

The A-scan device uses sound waves of low energy that permit the measurement to be made easily and quickly.

B Scan

The B scanner is similar to the A scanner in that low-energy sound waves are used, but its purpose is to produce an image of the eyeball on a special oscilloscope screen. The doctor may be unable to see the back of the eye because of the presence of a cataract, so the B scan is particularly important in ruling out serious eye problems such as retinal detachments and tumors. Sometimes photographs of the screen are taken so that the doctor has a permanent record that can be used for later comparisons.

K Readings

K readings are made by a keratometer. These measurements are of the curvature of the cornea (front surface) of the eye. The measurement is easy to make and does not require touching the eye. K readings are used for determining the proper contact lens a person requires as well as determining the necessary power of an implant lens in the event that an implant is being considered.

Fluorescein Angiography Test

A fluorescein eye test is used to determine the health of the rear (retina) of the eye. A fluorescein dye is given by injection or, in some cases, orally by pill and photographs are taken with a special flash camera. The fluorescein dye shows up brightly on the photograph and the doctor is then in a position to evaluate the circulation of the retina and any retinal problems that may exist.

External Eye Photographs

Often it is desirable to have a permanent record of what the front of the eye looks like before or after any surgery. In the case of an implant lens, the doctor may wish to have a record of its exact position. The camera used for this purpose is similar to a standard snapshot camera but may have a specialized lens and flash system.

Electrocardiogram

The electrical nature of the heartbeat permits the production of a graph of the beat of the heart, called an electrocardiogram or EKG. A doctor's training permits him to analyze the heartbeat for any problems or potential problems. It is important that electrocardiograms be done periodically so that comparisons can be used to reveal changes.

Prior to cataract surgery, an EKG ascertains if the patient's heart is functioning properly.

8

Visual Correction
After Surgery

Once you have had your cataract removed, there are several options for correcting your vision. They are spectacles (eyeglasses), hard contact lenses, soft contact lenses (daily and "permanent" types), and lens implants.

What you or your doctor chooses depends on your particular circumstances. For the moment, though, let us consider some general truths.

One is that you cannot wear glasses alone after cataract surgery if you have had only one cataract and the other eye sees well—unless you happen to be very, very nearsighted. The reason is that you would have double vision.

Suppose the eye that had the cataract operation has a thick spectacle lens in front of it, which magnifies the image. Suppose, too, that the other eye, which sees well and did not have a cataract, has a normal-size image. In most cases, everything you look at you would be seeing double, and the brain cannot fuse this into one image. So you can understand that wearing spectacle glasses following one cataract operation, when the other eye sees well, is usually not possible.

Either a contact lens or an implant must be used in the operated eye, or else one of the eyes must be blocked out with a patch of some kind. This is very important for you to understand. I venture to say that the most common question I get in my office is, "Doctor, why can't I just wear glasses after the operation? My aunt had cataract surgery and she wears glasses."

Well, your aunt may wear glasses. But either she had both eyes operated on or her other eye has a dense cataract and she does not see well enough through it to get double vision.

If you are sixty years of age or older, unless you have certain contraindications to implants such as severe diabetes, severe hypertension (high blood pressure), or bleeding tendencies, an implant should probably be your first choice. Once it is in, it does not have to be removed, cleaned, or taken care of in any special way.

Another option is to try a contact lens, knowing that if you cannot tolerate it, an implant can be put in later.

In fact, an implant can be put in anytime after you have had cataract surgery—even years or decades later.

Many of my patients who had cataract surgery ten or fifteen years ago are coming back for implants. They were unable to wear contacts for one reason or another and now want better vision than they are getting with spectacles.

Another point to remember is that contact lenses are not recommended for patients who live or work in dusty, polluted areas. Foreign-body sensations and even ulcers of the cornea can result if particles get under your contact lens.

The patient who works in a highly industrial, polluted area should therefore consider the alternative of the intraocular lens implant.

Given these general truths, let us examine each of the postoperative methods available to correct your vision.

Spectacles

Cataract glasses (see figure 11) are thick in most cases because they must reproduce the focusing power of the lens that had the cataract and that was removed.

If a person is going to have two cataract operations and his vision is not very critical postoperatively, he can wear spectacles afterward.

The problem with spectacles, though, is that central vision may be clear, although magnified, but when the patient looks to the side, his peripheral vision is quite blurred.

If a person leads a very sedentary life, this may not be a problem. But if he travels a lot, especially on public transportation, or certainly if he has to drive, cataract spectacles are no longer the treatment of choice.

Figure 12 is an approximation of what a patient sees with cataract spectacles. Notice that the center is clear but that the edges are extremely blurred. True, the patient can see clearly to the side by turning his head, and that is why you see elderly patients with thick glasses turning their heads every which way. They can only see someone standing next to them by turning around to face the person.

Contact Lenses

Whether one eye or both are operated on, the contact lens can be the patient's salvation. Contacts come in two kinds, hard and soft. In terms of vision, there is only a slight difference. Most patients get perfectly adequate results with the soft contact lens. And if a person has never worn contact lenses before, this is the lens to be used.

If a person is too infirm, or unable to learn how to put in a contact lens and take it out every day, there are specific types of contact lenses that can be left in, sometimes for months at a time, after which the patient returns to the ophthalmologist to have the lens cleaned and reinserted.

Unfortunately, only about 50 percent of contact lens wearers, in my experience, are able to tolerate the "permanent-wear" contact lens. Many elderly patients have somewhat dry eyes, and the contact lens, after being worn for a day, dries out and becomes irritating. This can lead to simple problems such as tearing (weeping) and redness, and even to complicated problems such as ulcers of the eye. If you are a permanent-contact-lens wearer, therefore, and your eye is chronically irritated and red, you must immediately go to see your ophthalmologist to make certain you are not developing some other complication.

Let us look more closely at the three types of contact lenses:

Hard Contact Lens This, of course, was the first type of contact lens to be developed, and it gives slightly better vision than the soft contact lens. It is made of a substance very similar to Plexiglas℗, is very thin, and although there is a foreign-body sensation when you first put it into your eye, after several hours or days this sensation disappears and you are usually unaware that the lens is there. It does require an adjustment period. The hard contact is fairly easy to insert and also fairly easy to remove. As I have said, if a patient has never worn contact lenses, I do not recommend the hard lens after surgery.

Daily-Wear Soft Contact Lens This contact lens feels like very soft rubber, but it is a synthetic material with a very high water content. When you first put this lens in your eye there is total comfort almost at once. There is no foreign-body sensation, and the vision is usually 20/20 or at least very close to it, if the eye is normal.

The lenses must be removed at night. They are put in a sterilizing solution while the wearer sleeps. The old days of boiling lenses are gone.

Putting the lens in the eye and taking it out is not a very complicated procedure, and anyone who has fairly nimble fingers and a fairly normal (not unusually small) eye can learn to wear daily-wear soft contact lenses.

Permanent-Wear Soft Contact Lenses These lenses are even higher in water content than the daily-wear soft contacts, and about half of cataract lens patients can tolerate them for several months at a time. Because these lenses remain in the eye for a long period of time, and deposits and secretions build up on them, vision is not usually quite as good as with the other two types of lenses.

Again, if you have a dry eye, or a tendency toward lid infections, these lenses are not recommended.

Lens Implant

In the early 1950s, Dr. Harold Ridley, a British ophthalmologist, observed that when splinters of Plexiglas were imbedded in pilots' eyes after airplane crashes, they remained inert and did not cause any foreign-body reaction. He theorized that this material could be used to make intraocular lenses, to replace contact lenses or spectacles.

In theory, Dr. Ridley was entirely correct. In practice, however, the Plexiglas lenses made at that time were not of sufficiently high quality for the human eye to retain them. Some of these lenses were rejected by the eyes because the edges were not polished adequately, or because the design of the lens was not yet perfected. But they were not rejected because of the Plexiglas.

When some of these lenses began to be rejected, the majority of eye surgeons abandoned the use of all intraocular lenses. But some, such as Cornelius Binkhorst and Peter Choyce in Europe, and Norman Jaffee, Miles Galin, and Henry Hirschman in this country, persisted with implants of various types. They found that these implants actually were safe and did give excellent results.

About ten years ago implants began to be used in increasing numbers in the United States. Since this was such a crucial area for the consumer, the Food and Drug Administration became involved. It set up rigid standards for the use of the implants and the reporting of any problems.

These rigid standards and reporting systems are still required today. There are now dozens of styles of intraocular implants, three of which I am personally responsible for (see figure 13), and all of which give excellent results in a high percentage of cases. Actually, the success rate is similar to the success rate of ordinary cataract surgery today.

You may have heard that implants are used only in very old people. This is no longer true. When we first began investigating implants, we put them only into patients aged seventy years and older. At that time we had only about a ten- or fifteen-year follow-up on those European lenses. If a seventy-year-old patient had problems with lenses, by the time he was eighty-five it would not be so serious, whereas if we had put the lenses into a fifty-year-old, he would have had problems at the age of sixty-five.

Fortunately, long-term problems have not shown up, and now we can put the lenses into patients fifty years of age and even younger, with a fairly good assurance that no problems will develop in these eyes in later years.

In my practice, I have even put these lenses into the eyes of some teenagers, who could not wear contact lenses because their corneas were deformed. In each case, the patient had a traumatic cataract in one eye.

Even these teenagers are doing fine, and I anticipate they will be able to live the rest of their lives with their implants.

There are various types and styles of implants, but the results are basically similar. Each has a slight advantage and it usually boils down to the implant that your particular surgeon is most comfortable using.

This is a highly technical area, and I would not recommend that, on the basis of reading some newspaper report, you recommend to your surgeon that he use either an anterior chamber implant, a posterior chamber implant, or any other specific kind. Let him (or her) decide this on the basis of his or her own experience.

As for results, the vision the patient gets with an implant is the closest to his normal physiological vision with his own lens.

The vision is usually corrected for middle distance. That is to say, you can see clearly at two to three feet. Distance vision is then corrected with *thin* spectacles which you do not always have to wear, but only, say, when driving.

Recently, the FDA has given permission for some ophthalmologists to use implants in certain infants who have cataracts. The safety and efficacy of these implants are finally being proved as they are monitored by government scientists.

Which would you choose—spectacles, contact lenses, or implants? After reading this chapter, you should be able to make this decision, with the help of your doctor.

9

Seeing or Suing
Your Doctor

Some people, after cataract surgery, think that if they cannot see their doctor, they should sue him. Since medical malpractice suits are a way of life today, it is something I should like to cover briefly in this chapter.

As I said very early in this book, the vast majority of ophthalmic surgeons are devoted, honest, competent, and caring. And remember that cataract surgery is about 95 percent successful. That means that about five out of every one hundred patients are going to have some kind of difficulty, no matter how good a surgeon is, and no matter how perfect the surgery was.

But that also means that ninety-five out of a hundred are going to get pretty much what they expected. So the odds are very much in your favor.

But suppose, just suppose, that you have had your operation and the world is still a dim blur. Your hopes for perfect vision were not realized. Naturally you are disappointed, even angry at your ophthalmologist—angry enough to sue him. Do you have grounds?

Answering the following questions will help you decide whether or not you should even entertain this course of action.

Did the ophthalmologist promise you perfect results? Or did he explain the small incidence of complications and state that you might have one? If he flatly said to you, "Don't worry, there won't be any problem," and did not explain any further, this may be considered lack of informed consent.

But you must be aware if you signed a form giving consent for surgery, the explanation of complications might have been contained in that form.

If no one accompanied you to the hospital, did the nurse read the consent form to you? Or if you were with a relative or friend, and were unable to read the form yourself, did that person read it to you? If you were able to read with your other eye, did you take the time to read the consent form before you signed it?

In any case, signing the consent form implied that you were familiar with the possible complications. That is basically the reason for having you sign one in the hospital, and usually in the doctor's office also.

For this reason, I believe it is very difficult for a patient to prove lack of informed consent today.

Another question to ask yourself if you think you should sue for malpractice is, "Did the doctor see me if and when I had complaints following the surgery, or did he make me wait a long time?" If you had a complication following surgery, that in itself does not constitute malpractice. However, if the doctor refused to see you, or was too busy to see you for a long period of time, this could be a serious point against him in a malpractice case.

Suppose, for example, you had the symptoms of a retinal detachment and called your surgeon and told him about this wall coming up from the ground. He then told you to come in immediately for an examination, made the diagnosis of the detachment, and sent you for repair. If then your vision was not restored, I do not believe this could be considered malpractice. (This of course is my opinion as a doctor. I am not a lawyer.)

On the other hand, if he said not to worry about this wall in front of you and told you to come in and see him in a couple of weeks, that would certainly be construed as improper medical practice.

The same thing would be true in reference to treating an infection, a hemorrhage, or some other complication following cataract surgery. The complication itself is not malpractice, but the refusal to treat, or a postponement of treatment, could be considered just that.

Another question you might ask yourself is, "Was the operation really necessary?" Certainly, if you had read this book, you would never have had an unnecessary operation. You would have known that unless your vision was seriously disturbed, affecting your way of life, surgery was not indicated in most instances.

If several doctors told you that you did not need an operation and one doctor did recommend surgery, and the eye had a complicated postoperative course, the loss of vision and the medical records of the other doctors could serve to prove that surgery was not necessary. But since this is really a matter of judgment on the part of the surgeon, it is not easy definitely to prove this point.

"Was my surgeon concerned about my complication?" is another question to ponder. Most surgeons with a 95 percent success rate are extremely disturbed if they have a patient with a postoperative complication, and even if they were to try to hide their disappointment and unhappiness from the patient, they could not.

But if a doctor dismisses your complication as one of those unfortunate instances and does not give you support, encouragement, and proper treatment, although these are not proofs of malpractice in any way, they certainly are responsible for many cases of medical malpractice lawsuits. It is for this reason that you must have good rapport with your ophthalmologist prior to surgery. It is for this reason that you should remain under the care of an ophthalmologist who knows you and has been treating you, and whose patients have told you they are satisfied with their surgical results.

It is my hope that after reading this book you will be better able to decide if, when, where, and how to have your cataract removed. It is my hope that this book will help you to see.

An important announcement has been made to all ophthalmologists at the time of the publication of this book.

The National Institutes of Health reported the results of a study of the effectiveness of laser treatment for senile macular degeneration (hardening of the arteries of the eye).

In this book I have consistently stated that there was no effective treatment for this disease. The purpose of the report of the National Institutes of Health was to alert ophthalmologists that a recent study has shown that, *if caught early,* certain types of macular degeneration are significantly improved with laser treatments, and the use of this treatment can prevent blindness in that eye. The emphasis is on early recognition and early treatment.

Every patient over the age of sixty must therefore be checked frequently for macular degeneration. Ideally, this should be done in the ophthalmologist's office several times a year. The test is called the Amsler Grid Test. The patient can, however, test himself by looking at the center of the Amsler Grid (figure 14). With first one eye covered and then the other, the patient should stare at the central white dot. If while staring at this dot any of the lines seem to be missing, or if the dot fades, this is a sign that macular degeneration may be starting in that eye and the patient should immediately contact his ophthalmologist. Any change in the patient's vision, particularly when looking at small print where straight lines seem to be slightly curved or fuzzy in the center, should also cause the patient to go to his ophthalmologist immediately.

Glossary

Amblyopia Poor vision in an eye in spite of the normal structure. It is usually due to suppression of that eye by the brain because the eye was turned in or out. It is sometimes called a lazy eye.

Aqueous Humor The fluid in the front portion of the eye in front of the lens. The nutrients in this fluid nourish the structures of the eye that do not have blood vessels, that is, the cornea and the lens.

Cataract A clouding of the lens resulting in partial to complete loss of vision.

Cataractogenic Anything that can cause a cataract. Certain medications, such as cortisone, when taken in large doses over a long period of time, have been implicated and should be used only under the strict and continual supervision of one's physician.

Congenital Conditions seen at birth. Cataracts can be congenital. Sometimes congenital conditions are hereditary, that is, passed down from generation to generation. Other times they are the result of an infection, such as German measles, in the pregnant mother.

Cornea A clear window in the very front of the eye that not only allows light to pass through but also helps to focus the light.

Corneal Graft   A small button removed from a donor eye.

Cryoextraction   Removal of a cataract by lifting it out with a cryogenic (freezing) probe.

Cryogenic   Cryo means cold. A cryogenic probe is one that gets cold enough to freeze to the cataract, simplifying its removal.

Cryoprobe   A freezing probe that adheres to a cataract firmly so that the cataract can be removed without spilling any of the contents of the cataract back into the eye.

Crystalline Lens   The natural lens of the eye. When it becomes cloudy, it is called a cataract.

Diabetes   A disease, basically of the pancreas, which after many years can affect the eyesight.

Diabetic Retinopathy   The name of the condition when diabetes affects the retina of the eye.

Edema   The swelling due to an accumulation of fluid in the eye, which can be seen in the cornea and the macula.

Emmetropia   Normal clear vision without the help of glasses or contact lenses.

Endothelial Cells   The cells that line the back of the cornea. Healthy cells in proper quantity are required for corneal transparency.

Endothelial Dystrophy   Degeneration of the cells lining the internal surface of the cornea. This condition is usually hereditary.

Extracapsular Cataract Surgery   A technique of surgery whereby the front capsule is opened at the time of surgery and the meat of the cataract is exposed. The eye is opened somewhat less than with an intracapsular extraction—about three-eighths of the way around—and the cataract is expressed, or pushed out of the eye. The remnants of the cataract are then vacuumed out with a small probe. The hospitalization for this operation is anywhere from one day to three days and the recuperation is usually from two to four weeks before full activities can be resumed. It is a safe and effective way of removing cataracts.

Fovea The center of the part of the eye used for fine vision. *See* MACULA.

Glaucoma An increase of the normal pressure inside the eye leading to pressure on the optic nerve and progressive loss of side vision. It is painless and often undetected by the patient in chronic cases. In an acute attack, the pain can be extremely severe.

Hypermature Cataract One that is swollen and filled with fluid and could conceivably rupture, causing acute pain, discomfort, and possible permanent loss of vision.

Hyperopia Farsightedness, a condition wherein a patient may require glasses for close work as well as for distance viewing.

Hypertensive Retinopathy The name of the condition when high blood pressure affects the retina.

Implant A man-made plastic lens inserted into the eye either at or after cataract surgery to replace the focusing power of the cloudy lens (cataract), which has been removed surgically.

Infrared Waves Long, low-frequency waves that are invisible to the human eye but can sometimes be felt as heat.

Intracapsular Cataract Surgery The technique whereby the entire cataract is removed *within* its capsule. It requires a large incision (halfway around the front of the eye) and anywhere from six to ten sutures, depending on the surgeon. The cataract is usually removed with a cryoprobe. It is a safe and effective method of removing cataracts, with a recuperation period of approximately four to six days in the hospital followed by about a month of convalescence before full activities can be resumed.

Iris The colored portion of the eye. It can open or close to regulate the amount of light that comes in.

Laser An acronym for Light Amplification by Stimulated Emission of Radiation. It is a very powerful beam of light that is capable of burning or destroying tissues where it is focused. It is used in ophthalmology for the treatment of retinal detachment and now, in its newest form, for opening up the posterior capsule after surgery. This latest laser was developed by Dr. Daniele Aron-Rosa in Paris.

Lens *See* CRYSTALLINE LENS.

Macula The part of the retina concerned with fine vision and used for reading, sewing, etc. The center of the macula, the area of the most critical vision, is called the fovea.

Macular Degeneration Commonly referred to as hardening of the arteries of the eye. It significantly reduces central reading vision. There is no treatment for it at present.

Macular Edema A condition following cataract surgery that reduces vision in most cases temporarily and in a very few cases permanently. The cause is unknown.

Millimeter Approximately one fortieth of an inch.

Myopia Nearsightedness, usually associated with a certain amount of stretching of the eye. The patient can see clearly up close without glasses, but in the distance his vision is blurred.

Ophthalmologist An ophthalmologist is a medical doctor. He has graduated from college and from medical school, taken an internship in general medicine, and then taken a specialty residency for an additional three years. He is able to provide complete eye care, including refraction for eyeglasses, treatment of eye diseases, and surgery of the eye.

Optician An optician is someone trained in the art of *making* lenses and glasses as well as contact lenses. He is trained to fill the prescription of an ophthalmologist or an optometrist. He may not diagnose diseases or refractive conditions of the eye.

Optometrist An optometrist is a licensed practitioner in

the art of *prescribing* glasses and contact lenses. He does not have a medical degree and is not able to diagnose general medical conditions.

Phacoemulsification A method for breaking up a cataract with an ultrasonic needle and vacuuming it out at the same time. It is a form of extracapsular extraction in that part of the capsule remains. Since there is only one suture, the rehabilitation is usually one day in the hospital after which the patient can resume most normal activities. It is a safe and effective means of removing a cataract.

Photophobia Sensitivity to light.

Posterior Capsule The back layer of a cataract, which is usually clear but sometimes clouds after cataract surgery. It can be opened with a very minor surgical procedure or with the new Aron-Rosa laser.

Presbyopia The condition wherein a patient who was once able to see at close range loses that ability and must wear reading glasses. This usually occurs some time after the age of forty to forty-five years.

Pupil The black hole in the center of the iris that resembles the hole in a doughnut. It is black because no light is reflected back from the bottom of a deep well and the center looks black.

Retina The nerve layer of the eye. It has cells that are sensitive to light. When light falls on the retina, an electrical impulse is conducted from the eye to the brain and the person sees.

Retinal Detachment A sight-threatening condition in which the retina becomes loose from its attachment and peels forward toward the vitreous. It can usually be corrected surgically if repaired early enough. Otherwise the delicate retinal cells will die.

Retinal Hole A small defect in the retina that can in many instances lead to retinal detachment. Diagnosis of the hole before a detachment is produced allows the surgeon to treat the hole very simply with freezing. Freezing over the hole creates an inflammation that seals the hole and prevents a retinal detachment.

Ripe Cataract The term that was used to describe a cataract that had hardened sufficiently to be easily pushed out of the eye in one piece, leaving little debris behind. With modern methods of cataract surgery, it is not necessary to wait for the lens to ripen, or harden.

Sclera The white of the eye. It completely surrounds the eyeball except in the very front of the eye where the sclera becomes totally clear and is called the cornea.

Suture Commonly known as a "stitch." It is a fine strand of fiber used by the surgeon to close an incision. Cataract sutures are sometimes left in place and sometimes removed, depending on the type of suture. The common sutures used are silk or nylon or absorbable sutures such as fine catgut.

Trachea The tube leading from the throat to the lungs.

Ultrasonic A frequency higher than that which can be heard by the human ear (approximately ten thousand cycles). Any instrument that is vibrating at more than ten thousand cycles (vibrations per second) is considered ultrasonic.

Ultraviolet Rays High-frequency, very short light waves, mostly invisible to the human eye.

Vitrectomy Surgical removal of the vitreous. In some cases, this procedure is used to treat severe eye infections.

Vitreous The clear jelly that fills all the space behind the lens; in other words, most of the eye.

Vitreous Hemorrhage Bleeding into the jelly of the eye, usually associated with long-standing diabetes. The blood sometimes clears, but has a tendency to recur.

Zonules Ligaments that hold the crystalline lens in place and which, by action of the internal muscles of the eye, change the shape of the lens to bring an object into focus.

List of Local Ophthalmology
Associations and Resources

Alabama

Alabama Academy of Ophthalmology
1720 Eighth Avenue S.
Birmingham, AL 35233

Alaska

No listing available

Arizona

Arizona Ophthalmological Society
1951 Riviera Drive
Lake Havasu City, AZ 86403

Phoenix Ophthalmological Society
13660 N. 94th Drive
Peoria, AZ 85345

Arkansas

Arkansas Medical Society, Eye Section
P. O. Box 908
Fayetteville, AR 72701

California

California Association of Ophthalmology
6367 Alvarado Court, Suite 101
San Diego, CA 92120

California Medical Association, Ophthalmology Section
5333 Hollister Avenue
Santa Barbara, CA 93111

Alta California Ophthalmological Society
3939 J Street
Sacramento, CA 95819

Los Angeles Society of Ophthalmology
450 N. Bedford Drive, Suite 101
Beverly Hills, CA 90210

Peninsula Eye Society
881 Fremont Avenue
Los Altos, CA 94022

Pacific Coast Oto-Ophthalmological Society
2122 W. Third Street
Los Angeles, CA 90057

San Diego Academy of Ophthalmology
317 North El Camino Real, Suite 402
Encinitas, CA 92024

San Francisco Ophthalmological Round Table
490 Post Street
San Francisco, CA 94108

Tri-County Society of Ophthalmology
1535 West Merced
West Covina, CA 91790

Colorado

Colorado Ophthalmological Society
4545 East Ninth Avenue
Denver, CO 80220

Connecticut

Connecticut Society of Eye Physicians
477 South Broad Street
Meriden, CT 06450

Delaware

Delaware Academy of Ophthalmology
521 Dupont Highway
Milford, DE 19963

District of Columbia

Medical Society of the District of Columbia
Section of Ophthalmology
600 Hillwood Avenue
Falls Church, VA 22042

Florida

Florida Society of Ophthalmology
421 Park Avenue N.
Winter Park, FL 32789

Miami Ophthalmological Society
1100 NE 163rd Street
North Miami Beach, FL 33162

Georgia

Atlanta Ophthalmological Society
490 Peachtree Street, Suite 331
Atlanta, GA 30338

Georgia Society of Ophthalmology
653 Cherokee Street
Marietta, GA 30060

Hawaii

Hawaii Ophthalmological Society
320 Ward Avenue
Honolulu, HI 96814

Idaho

Idaho Society of Ophthalmology
921 Fifth Avenue
Sandpoint, ID 83864

Illinois

Illinois Association of Ophthalmology
1702 Washington Street
Waukegan, IL 60085

Illinois Society of Ophthalmology and Otolaryngology
200 South College Street
Danville, IL 60183

Rock River Valley Ophthalmology Association
1211 Talcott Building
Rockford, IL 61101

Indiana

Indiana Academy of Ophthalmology
1646 45th Avenue
Munster, IN 46321

Indianapolis Ophthalmological and Otolaryngological
Society
5506 East 16th Street
Indianapolis, IN 46218

Iowa

Iowa Academy of Ophthalmology
c/o Department of Ophthalmology
University Hospitals
Iowa City, IA 52240

Quad City Ophthalmological Society
Suite 512, Davenport Bank Building
Davenport, IA 52801

Kansas

Kansas City Society of Ophthalmology and
Otolaryngology
2928 Main Street, Suite 230
Kansas City, KS 64108

Kansas State Medical Society, Section of
Ophthalmology
3333 E. Central, Suite 722
Wichita, KS 67208

Kentucky

Kentucky Academy of Eye Physicians and Surgeons
4001 Dutchmans Lane
Louisville, KY 40207

Northern Kentucky Eye, Ear, Nose, and Throat Society
802 Scott Street
Covington, KY 41011

Louisville Academy of Ophthalmology
4001 Dutchmans Lane
Louisville, KY 40207

Louisiana

Louisiana Ophthalmology Association
9104 Quine Street
New Orleans, LA 70118

New Orleans Academy of Ophthalmology
Maison Blanche Building, 921 Canal Street
New Orleans, LA 70112

Maine

Maine Society of Eye Physicians and Surgeons
325A Kennedy Memorial Drive
Waterville, ME 05901

Maryland

Maryland Academy of Ophthalmology
3450 Fort Meade Road, Suite 200
Laurel, MD 20810

Maryland Ophthalmological Society
14 West Mount Vernon Place
Baltimore, MD 21201

Massachusetts

Massachusetts Society of Eye Physicians and Surgeons
280 Washington Street
Brighton, MA 02135

Michigan

Michigan Ophthalmological Society
3535 West 18 Mile Road
Royal Oak, MI 48072

Detroit Ophthalmological Society
6001 West Outer Drive
Detroit, MI 48239

Saginaw Valley Academy of Ophthalmology and
Otolaryngology
5481 Colony Drive North
Saginaw, MI 48603

Minnesota

Minnesota Association of Ophthalmology and
Otolaryngology
220 Doctors Professional Building
280 Smith Avenue N.
St. Paul, MN 55102

Minnesota Academy of Ophthalmology and
Otolaryngology
Central Medical Building, Suite 414
St. Paul, MN 55104

Mississippi

Mississippi Eye, Ear, Nose, and Throat Association
882 Lakeland Drive
Jackson, MS 39201

Jackson Ophthalmological Society
St. Dominic's Medical Offices
971 Lakeland Drive
Jackson, MS 39201

Missouri

Missouri Ophthalmological Society
1321 Village Drive
St. Joseph, MO 64506

Kansas City Society of Ophthalmology and
Otolaryngology
Jackson County Medical Society
3036 Gillham Road
Kansas City, MO 64108

St. Louis Ophthalmological Society
211 N. Meramec
St. Louis, MO 63105

Montana

Montana Academy of Ophthalmology and
Otolaryngology
2000 Clark Street
Miles City, MT 59301

Nebraska

Nebraska Academy of Ophthalmology
600 N. Cotner Boulevard
Lincoln, NE 68505

Omaha Ophthalmological Society
234 Doctors Building, 4239 Farnam
Omaha, NE 68102

Nevada

Las Vegas Ophthalmological Society
3196 S. Maryland Parkway
Las Vegas, NV 89109

New Hampshire

New Hampshire Society of Eye Physicians and Surgeons
4 Park Street
Concord, NH 03301

New Jersey

New Jersey Academy of Ophthalmology and
Otolaryngology
15 S. Ninth Street
Newark, NJ 07107

New Mexico

New Mexico Association of Ophthalmology
P. O. Drawer DD
Espanola, NM 87533

New Mexico Ophthalmological Society
465 St. Michaels Drive
Santa Fe, NM 87501

New York

New York Academy of Medicine, Section of
Ophthalmology
635 West 165th Street
New York, NY 10032

New York Society for Clinical Ophthalmology
146 E. 71st Street
New York, NY 10021

New York State Medical Society, Section of
Ophthalmology
677 Madison Avenue
New York, NY 10021

New York State Ophthalmological Society
667 Madison Avenue
New York, NY 10021

Alumni Association of the New York Eye and Ear
Infirmary
635 West 165th Street
New York, NY 10032

Brooklyn Ophthalmological Society
7423 Shore Road
Brooklyn, NY 11229

Buffalo Ophthalmological Club
3834 Delaware Avenue
Kenmore, NY 14217

Eastern New York Eye, Ear, Nose and Throat
Association
Albany Medical Center Hospital
Albany, NY 12208

Long Island Ophthalmological Society
North Shore
Manhasset, NY 11030

Nassau Academy of Medicine, Section of
Ophthalmology
4277 Hempstead Turnpike
Bethpage, NY 11714

Rochester Ophthalmological Society
277 Alexander Street
Rochester, NY 14607

Westchester County Medical Society
Section of Ophthalmology
35 Adams Street
Bedford Hills, NY 10507

North Carolina

North Carolina Society of Ophthalmology
3410 Executive Drive
Raleigh, NC 27609

North Dakota

North Dakota Academy of Ophthalmology and
Otolaryngology
1605 E. Capitol Avenue
Bismarck, ND 58501

Ohio

Ohio Ophthalmological Society
363 E. Town Street
Columbus, OH 43215

Cincinnati Society of Ophthalmology
7815 Beechmont Avenue
Cincinnati, OH 45230

Cleveland Ophthalmological Society
Cleveland Metropolitan General Hospital
3395 Scranton Road
Cleveland, OH 44109

Toledo Ophthalmological Society
3103 Executive Parkway
Toledo, OH 43606

Oklahoma

Oklahoma State Society of Ophthalmologists
Dean A. McGee Eye Institute
Oklahoma City, OK 73104

Oregon

Oregon Academy of Ophthalmology
421 High Street
Oregon City, OR 97045

Pennsylvania

Pennsylvania Academy of Ophthalmology and
Otolaryngology
Department of Medical Education, Wills Eye Hospital
Philadelphia, PA 19107

Ophthalmic Club of Philadelphia
406 Cooper Street
Camden, NJ 19151

Philadelphia College of Physicians
Section of Ophthalmology
Wills Eye Hospital
Philadelphia, PA 19107

Pittsburgh Ophthalmological Society
1420 Center Street
Pittsburgh, PA 15235

Reading Eye, Ear, Nose and Throat Society
301 S. Seventh Avenue
West Reading, PA 19611

Wills Eye Hospital Society
Suite 135, Lankenau Hospital
Philadelphia, PA 19151

Rhode Island

Rhode Island Ophthalmological Society
110 Lockwood
Providence, RI 02886

South Carolina

South Carolina Society of Ophthalmology and
Otolaryngology
397 Serpentine Drive
Spartanburg, SC 29303

Charleston Ophthalmological Society
112 Fairfield Office Park
Charleston, SC 29407

South Dakota

South Dakota Academy of Ophthalmology and
Otolaryngology
2727 South Kiwanis Avenue
Sioux Falls, SD 57105

Tennessee

Tennessee State Academy of Ophthalmology
Blount Professional Building No. 3
Knoxville, TN 37920

Knoxville Society of Ophthalmology
Suite 806, 939 Emerald Avenue
Knoxville, TN 37917

Memphis Society of Ophthalmology
4646 Poplar Avenue
Memphis, TN 38105

Nashville Academy of Ophthalmology and
Otolaryngology
300 25th Avenue N.
Nashville, TN 37203

Texas

Texas Ophthalmological Association
8210 Walnut Hill Lane
Dallas, TX 75231

Texas Society of Ophthalmology and Otolaryngology
902 Frostwood, Suite 179
Houston, TX 77024

Austin Ophthalmological Association
1020 West 34th Street
Austin, TX 78705

Houston Ophthalmological Society
1100 Hermann Professional Building
Houston, TX 77030

San Antonio Society of Ophthalmology and
Otolaryngology
1005 Nix Professional Building
San Antonio, TX 79205

Utah

Utah Ophthalmological Society
508 E.S. Temple Street
Salt Lake City, UT 84102

Vermont

Vermont Ophthalmological Society
254 Stratton Road
Rutland, VT 05701

Virginia

Northern Virginia Academy of Ophthalmology
121 N. Washington Street
Alexandria, VA 22314

Virginia Society of Ophthalmology and Otolaryngology
Staunton Medical Center
Staunton, VA 24401

Lynchburg Ophthalmological Society
2319 Atherhold Road
Lynchburg, VA 24501

Tidewater Eye Society
705 Medical Tower
Norfolk, VA 23507

Washington

Washington State Academy of Ophthalmology
16110 Eighth Avenue SW, Suite B2
Seattle, WA 98166

Washington State Medical Association
1300 116th Street NE
Bellevue, WA 98004

West Virginia

West Virginia Academy of Ophthalmology and
Otolaryngology
Frederick and Woodland Streets
Bluefield, WV 24701

Wisconsin

Wisconsin State Medical Society
850 Elm Grove Road
Elm Grove, WI 53122

Milwaukee Ophthalmological Society
2400 South 90th Street
West Allis, WI 53227

Wyoming

No listing available

Index

Illustrations are represented by figure numbers.

About the Author

Dr. Charles D. Kelman's breakthrough techniques and his inventions of machines and instruments to aid the surgeon in cataract surgery revolutionized methods that had been employed for two hundred years and have earned him an international reputation as one of the world's leading cataract surgeons as well as a place in the history of the medical profession.

In 1961, Dr. Kelman invented an electric cryogenic (freezing) probe that replaced forceps as a means of removing lenses that had developed cataracts.

Two years later, he began development of an ultrasonic probe, vibrating at a rate of forty thousand cycles, to dissolve, emulsify, and remove cataracts. The process is called phacoemulsification.

With the Kelman method, patients suffer less discomfort and resume their normal activities on the day following their operation, whereas the traditional operation means a convalescence of up to six weeks.

Dr. Kelman also is responsible for innovative designs of lens implants, which eliminate, in most cases, the need for thick glasses after cataract surgery.

Because Dr. Kelman's phacoemulsification technique has completely changed the world of cataract surgery, he is listed in *Who's Who in the World* as well as in *Who's Who in America*. Among other honors, he received the prestigious American Academy Achievement Award in 1969. (Among the prior recipients in medicine were Drs. Salk, Cooley, and De Bakey.)

Dr. Kelman, twice nominated for Inventor of the Year, is a fellow of the American Academy of Ophthalmology and the author of more than fifty articles, publications, and books. He has taught his technique to physicians who use it around the globe, in more than fifteen countries.

In addition to his private practice in New York City, Dr. Kelman is professor of ophthalmology at New York Medical College and chairman of the department of ophthalmology at Lydia Hall Hospital, Freeport, New York. Because of the heavy demands for his time, Dr. Kelman commutes between sites by helicopter, which he pilots himself.